SECRETS OF CRYSTALS

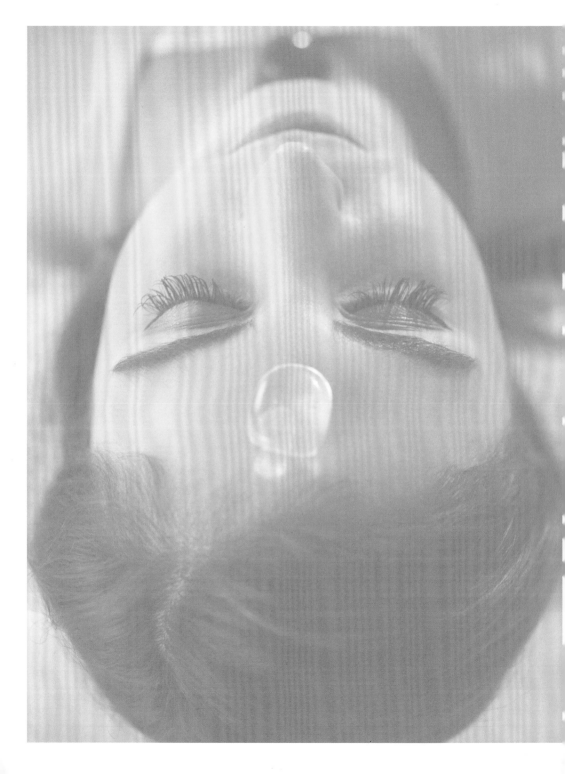

SECRETS OF
CRYSTALS

JENNIE HARDING

IVY PRESS

First published in the UK and North America in 2018 by
Ivy Press
An imprint of The Quarto Group
The Old Brewery, 6 Blundell Street
London N7 9BH, United Kingdom
T (0)20 7700 6700 **F** (0)20 7700 8066
www.QuartoKnows.com

British Library Cataloguing-in-Publication Data
A catalogue record for this book is available from the British Library

ISBN: 978-1-78240-572-6

This book was conceived, designed and produced by
Ivy Press
58 West Street, Brighton BN1 2RA, United Kingdom

Publisher: Susan Kelly
Creative Director: Michael Whitehead
Editorial Director: Tom Kitch
Art Director: James Lawrence
Project Editor: Elizabeth Clinton
Designer: Ginny Zeal
Illustrator: Nicky Ackland-Snow
Photographer: Neal Grundy
Model: Joe Menzies
Editorial Assistant: Niamh Jones

Printed in China

10 9 8 7 6 5 4 3 2 1

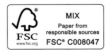

Note from the publisher
Information given in this book is not intended to be taken as a
replacement for medical advice. Any person with a condition
requiring medical attention should consult a qualified medical
practitioner or therapist.

Cover image: Shutterstock/Aleksandrov Ilia

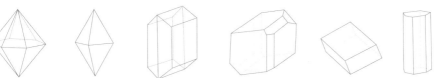

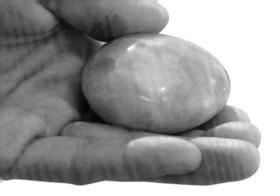

HOW TO USE THIS BOOK

You hold in your hands a personal guide to the world of crystal energy healing. This book will take you on a fascinating journey to discover the origins of crystals, how they are formed, and how to use them in your life to enhance your well-being. Crystals are beautiful gifts from Mother Earth, coming in many different shapes, sizes, and colors. Collecting crystals can become a life-long passion; it can also be a self-healing journey. By learning more about the crystals you are drawn to, you will feel connected to the planet in a deeper and more meaningful way. As you appreciate the miraculous processes that have, over millions of years, created the crystals that you collect, you will begin to appreciate their many beautiful qualities. In this book we will cover several aspects of the world of crystals; enjoy exploring it. The more you bring crystals into your life, the more you will experience their energy and their healing presence, and the more your relationship to the Earth will be deepened and transformed.

Important Notice

The claims in this book have been sincerely made, but neither the publisher or author can be held responsible for any claim or belief described. Please be aware that although crystals can be used for their energetic effects, they are not intended to be a substitute for any medical, hospital, or psychiatric treatment.

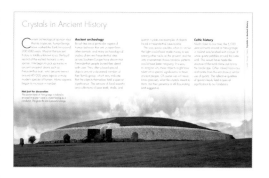

Understanding

Secrets of Crystals *introduces you to the geology of crystals and their uses throughout history.*

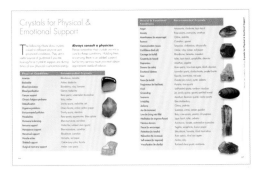

References

Tables outline the qualities and energetic effects of crystals to aid your selection.

Routines

Simple steps guide you through using and looking after your collection.

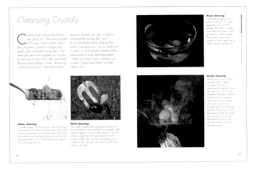

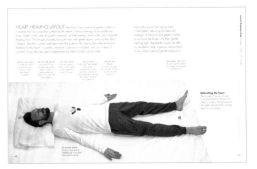

Crystal layouts

Practical visual guides explain how to use crystals to enhance your well-being.

Directory

An extensive index of crystals tells you what makes each one special and how to use them for their healing benefits.

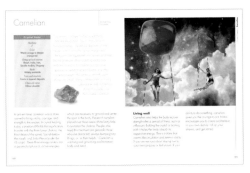

Introduction

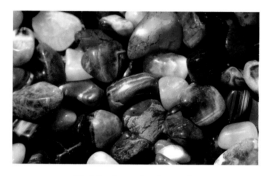

Multicolored minerals

Crystals occur in endless shades, shapes, and sizes; they are fascinating objects to collect.

Crystals are minerals that melted and fused themselves together inside the Earth at incredibly hot temperatures; over time, through countless cycles of heating and cooling, chemical reactions took place forming beautiful mineral structures. Crystals are found in caves or fissures deep in the Earth's crust, or lie buried in the ground until they are extracted. It is amazing to think that any piece of crystal you pick up has taken millions of years to form—and now you have it in your hand.

The appeal of crystals

There are a variety of reasons why crystals attract attention. They are lovely natural objects that sparkle or reflect light in different colors. There is something about them that makes you want to touch them, to pick them up and hold them, turn them to the light and see how they react. They are "moreish" too: once you start a collection you will find yourself adding to it all the time. Crystal healers say that you are drawn to crystals that are right for you—look at a tray of stones of the same type and you tend to find there is one that "calls" to you.

Reactions to crystals are purely instinctive. This is what makes collecting them so fun—it's a totally individual choice. Some people are drawn to collect really large crystals (if they can afford them; pieces like this tend to be very expensive) and other people prefer to have smaller crystals around, not just because of cost but because they like variety. There are no rules here: simply follow your instinct, trust your intuition, and the most beneficial crystals will find their way into your collection. Whether you are interested in crystals for their beauty, color, shape, or energetic qualities, they will always add a unique dimension to your life.

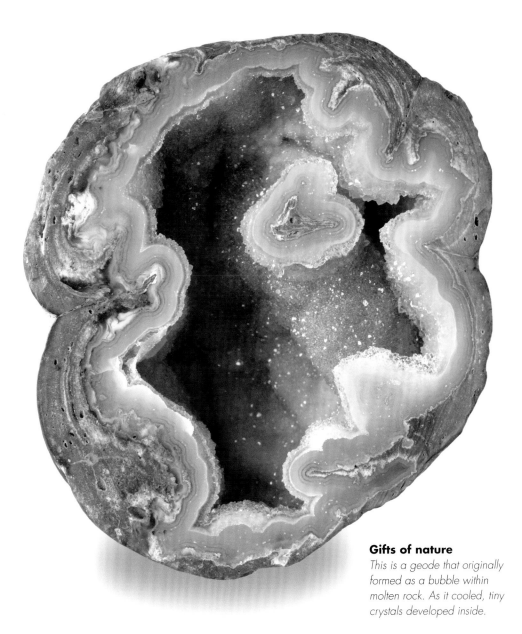

Gifts of nature
This is a geode that originally formed as a bubble within molten rock. As it cooled, tiny crystals developed inside.

THE GEOLOGY OF CRYSTALS

Crystals are created by incredible processes and cycles within the earth. In this chapter you will learn about the different kinds of crystals and their qualities, and how they need to be handled. Crystals are amazing things and some of their characteristics may surprise you. Understanding the relationship between crystals and the Earth helps you to appreciate the unique qualities of these minerals and how precious they truly are.

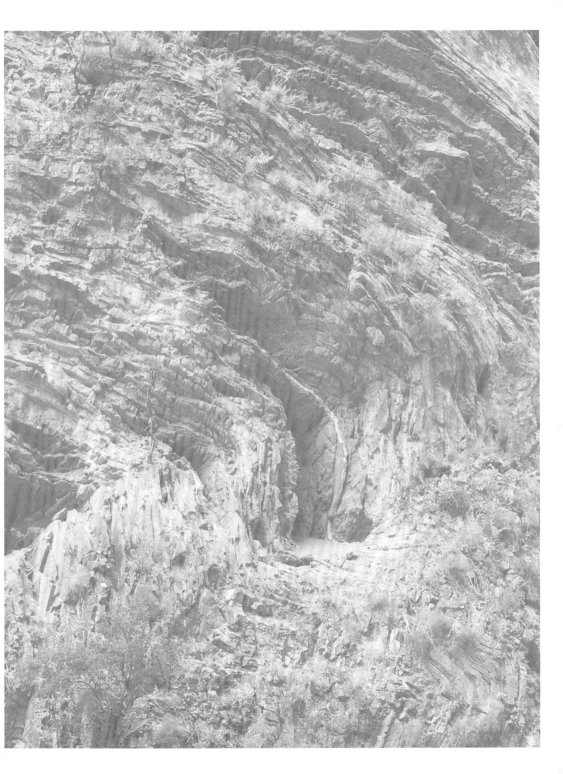

Introduction to an Evolving Earth

We speak of "solid ground," and it's easy to imagine the Earth that way: as constant and static. Unless we happen to live in an earthquake zone, we could be forgiven for thinking that the planet under our feet does not change. There is something very stabilizing and comforting about walking on the Earth, especially barefoot—a feeling of connection with a supremely strong and reassuring presence.

In fact, the Earth under our feet is a powerhouse of giant cycles, most of which pass us by. Volcanic eruptions are an occasional visual and physical reminder that the Earth is raging with inner fire. Changes are always happening; they simply do so extremely slowly. The timescales of the Earth are in millions of years with the planet itself estimated to be about 4.6 billion years old. In our planet's lifetime, endless cycles of heating, squeezing, and compressing the rocks that make up the Earth's crust has led to the formation of crystals, gems, metals, and other precious minerals.

Continental drift

Millions of years ago the raised parts of Earth's land mass did not look anything like the map of the world we see today. Continents have shifted, bumped into each other, pushed each other aside. Ancient oceans have come and gone, their beds dried out in layers, compressed and squeezed into rocks. The Himalayas, the highest mountain range on Earth, is made up of limestone rock layers; it used to be an ancient seabed, and over millions of years these layers of rock have been pushed up to form mountains.

It takes all this time for crystals to form; they are part of our planet's endless changes. When you buy a crystal, take time to think about the countless processes that have brought it to you, now, to hold.

Earth power
The intense heat of a volcanic eruption is able to melt rock so that it runs out onto the Earth's surface like a river.

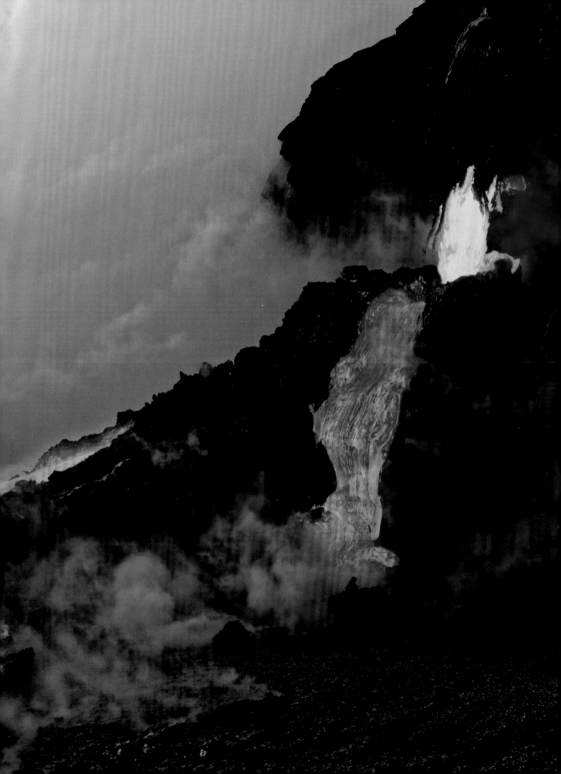

THE STRUCTURE OF THE EARTH

The Earth was formed billions of years ago as our solar system formed out of vast clouds of gas and cosmic dust, generated by the deaths of other stars. The Earth is structured in layers that constantly interact with each other over time; the intense heat within our planet fuels countless chemical reactions between elements, leading to the formation of mineral compounds, rocks, and, eventually, crystals.

The crust

The outer layer of the Earth, which we walk on, is the crust. It ranges from 3 to 44 miles (5 to 70 kilometers) thick; the thinnest parts are the beds of the oceans, while the continents that make up the land masses we occupy are thicker, in some places rising up into mountains. Many rocks making up the Earth's crust have been dated to around 100 million years old, showing that the crust is a "young" part of the Earth's structure because it is constantly being reformed over time. The crust is divided into tectonic plates, which are constantly pushing against each other and moving over the inner layers.

The mantle

The next layer is the mantle, extending to almost 1,900 miles (3,000 kilometers) deep; it is the thickest layer of the Earth. The mantle is the source of many silicate rocks, including quartz. Extremely high temperatures within the mantle cause expansion and movement of magma (molten rock) along the tectonic plates.

The core

The center of the Earth is the core. It is made up of extremely dense heavy elements such as nickel and iron. When the Earth started to form, the heavier weight of these elements drove them into the center of the planet. The core is made up of a molten outer layer and an inner layer containing precious metals such as gold and platinum. The iron in the Earth's core is highly magnetic and is the source of the Earth's magnetic field.

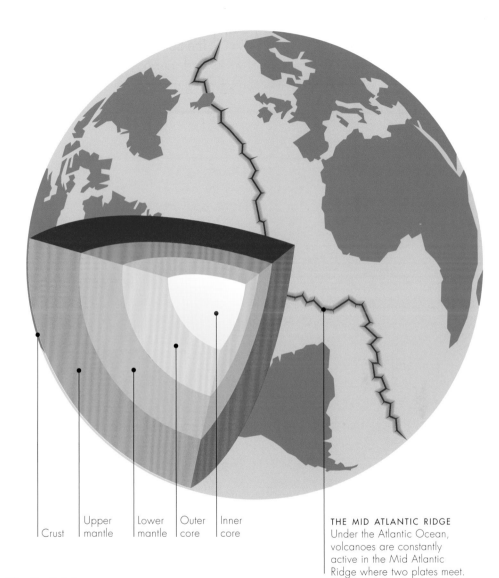

| Crust | Upper mantle | Lower mantle | Outer core | Inner core |

THE MID ATLANTIC RIDGE
Under the Atlantic Ocean,
volcanoes are constantly
active in the Mid Atlantic
Ridge where two plates meet.

The Earth's layers
The Earth is made up of three concentric layers,
the crust, the mantle, and the core. The mantle is
often split into the upper and lower mantle and
the core into the outer and inner core.

15

How Crystals Form

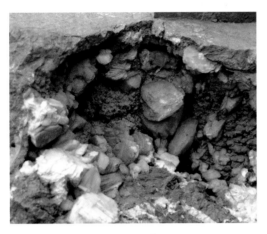

Layer upon layer
Within the Earth's crust, minerals and crystals lie on top of each other, squeezed and shaped in countless ways.

It is estimated that more than 2,500 different mineral compounds exist, including all kinds of crystals, and precious and semi-precious stones. All of them have formed due to individual chemical reactions between elements present in rock layers, sometimes through reactions with boiling hot magma, processes of heating and cooling over time, or the formation of "bubbles" in liquid rock enabling space for crystals to form.

Here are some examples of common crystals with details of their formation.

Calcite

Calcite is one of the most common minerals: calcium carbonate. It is a crystallization of limestone, a sedimentary rock—that is, one made up of the shells of dead marine organisms from ancient oceans. Calcite tends to be opaque rather than transparent, but sometimes examples with tiny clear crystals can be found. Calcite occurs in many colors, for example, cream (sometimes called honey calcite), blue, green, or orange. The colors are influenced by the chemical elements present in the surrounding rocks.

Quartz

Quartz, or silicon dioxide, is produced in rocks rich in the element silica, as they harden during a cooling phase. If water is present, as in hydrothermal vents, (deep cracks in the Earth's crust) over time, chemical reactions between silica and oxygen encourage the formation of six-sided crystal points. Most quartz is clear; different colored varieties are formed when other minerals are present. Amethyst (purple quartz) arises when iron combines with the silica/oxygen chemical reaction; rose quartz forms when elements such as titanium, iron, or manganese are present.

Jasper

Jasper forms out of chemical reactions between very fine volcanic ash or particles of magma that settle onto sources of silica, creating a fine-grained texture in the stone. Depending on the particular chemistry of the environment, many different colors and patterns are generated. Jasper is opaque, but because it contains microcrystalline grains its surface can be polished to a mirror-smooth finish. The most common type is red jasper, rich in iron, but jasper can be streaked, mottled, or patterned in many different colors.

Mass formation
In this riverbed, layers of red jasper stretch as far as the eye can see.

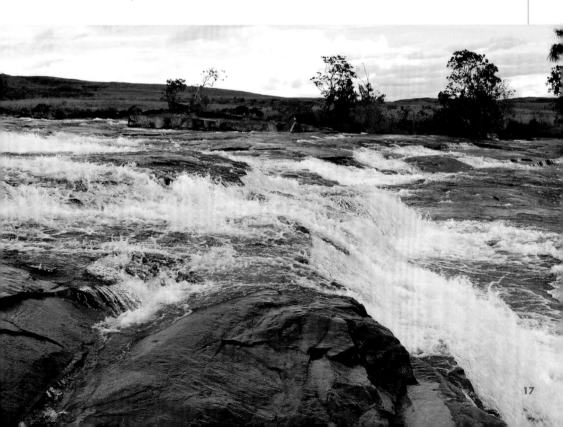

17

CRYSTAL GEOMETRY

Most crystals and precious gems, such as diamonds, rubies, and emeralds, are created by chemical reactions that influence their eventual shape. Different elements combine to create three-dimensional patterns as they cool down. It is the chemistry of this process that influences the structure that crystals take. Some end up quite symmetrical, appearing in vertical planes or triangular pyramid shapes; others form more cubic shapes. Temperature, pressure, and the rate of cooling as a crystal forms will influence the eventual shape. Crystals and gems conform to geometry in their configuration, as you will see from the diagrams opposite.

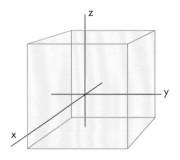

Geometrical axes

Axes are angles of formation that create different geometric shapes. A cube, for example, is made of three axes at 90 degrees to one another, creating a three-dimensional square.

Microcrystalline Quartz

Types of microcrystalline quartz such as carnelian, agates, chalcedony, jasper, and onyx form in a different way. They occur in banded layers or masses within rocks, and are composed of microscopic particles of quartz mixed with colored volcanic dust or mineral layers (sediments, such as mudrocks or sandstones). The colors arise from reactions between different chemical elements in the local environment. Microcrystalline quartz stones are colorful and polish up to a smooth surface, clearly showing any bands or lines in their construction; a common example is blue lace agate (below).

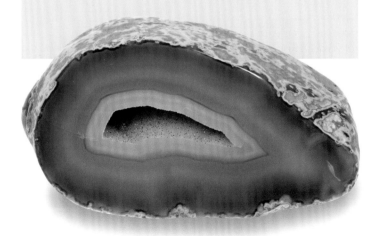

Crystal lattices

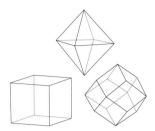

Cubic
Made up of three equal axes forming a cube. Examples are pyrite, diamond, and fluorite.

Hexagonal
Made up of four axes creating a six-fold symmetry. Examples are quartz, emerald, and aquamarine.

Tetragonal
This resembles two four-sided pyramids joined at the base. Examples are apophyllite and zircon.

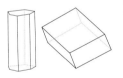

Orthorhombic
Made up of three axes at 90 degrees to each other. Examples are peridot and topaz.

Monoclinic
Made up of three unequal axes creating an elongated vertical shape. Examples are selenite and kunzite.

Triclinic
This is the most asymmetric shape. Examples are labradorite and turquoise.

Trigonal
This is an elongated lozenge shape. Examples are sapphire and tourmaline.

AMORPHOUS CRYSTALS

As well as crystals that follow geometric patterns as they form, there is a group that are called amorphous, which means "shapeless." These crystals are formed in unusual ways and have special uses in crystal healing.

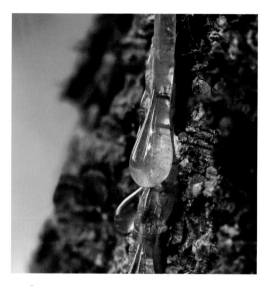

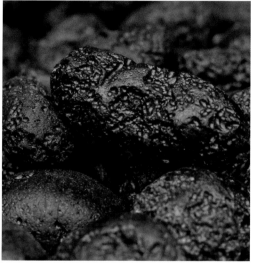

Amber

Most stones, minerals, and crystals are called inorganic minerals, meaning they are formed from basic chemical elements. Amber is called an organic mineral because it originally formed as a function of a living organism: a pine tree. Millions of years ago, resin—a sticky golden substance that oozes out of the bark of pine trees—dropped to the ground, sometimes picking up pollen grains, seeds, or even insects, and hardened over time, becoming fossilized. The beauty of amber lies in its smooth rounded shape, golden or orange-red color, and the variety of tiny objects it may contain, called inclusions.

Tektites

These are a kind of glass: meteorite glass. When a meteorite enters the Earth's atmosphere, it is heated to an incredibly high temperature. When the object actually hits the Earth, there are chemical reactions between meteorite fragments and the rocks and minerals in the Earth's soil. The meeting of the meteorite melts the rocks and soil into bubbly and irregular pieces of meteorite glass. One of the most famous tektites is called moldavite; this green volcanic glass formed after an ancient meteorite impact in southern Germany.

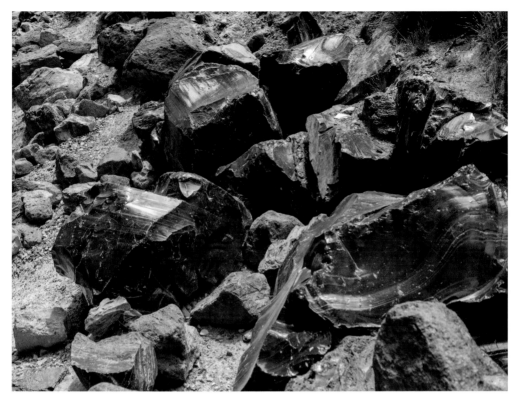

Obsidian

This is volcanic glass, formed where the silica-rich edges of a lava flow solidify into a shapeless mass. It is usually black or dark in color, but can have a misty or slightly speckled appearance, depending on other minerals present when it solidifies. Obsidian is hard but also brittle, meaning it can be cracked or shattered into very sharp-edged pieces. Ancient peoples made use of thin leaves of obsidian as razor-sharp knives, or shaped small pieces into arrowheads.

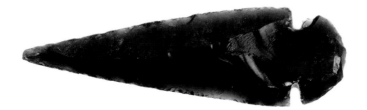

Crystal Hardness

Because crystals are minerals, it is easy to think that they are indestructible when actually this is not the case. The geometrical way that they form means that they contain planes—angles of formation—such as the vertical striations in selenite. If they are dropped, often they will shatter into smaller pieces along these planes. Crystals need to be stored safely and handled with care. Some are harder than others; the softer they are, the more vulnerable they are to damage.

The Mohs scale of hardness

In 1812 a German mineralogist called Friedrich Mohs created a scale to help identify different hardness in minerals. Hardness is a vital aspect in jewelry making; only the hardest stones such as topaz, corundum (ruby or sapphire), or diamond are able to be faceted, that is, cut into shapes that cause them to reflect even more light. Softer stones shatter, which is why they tend to be simply smoothed into rounded "cabochons" and polished for setting in jewelry. The Mohs scale runs from the softest at number 1 to the hardest at number 10.

Sometimes these values can be a surprise: for example, emerald, one of the most valuable of all gemstones, has only a 7 hardness. Emeralds are very difficult to facet without shattering; the stones are oiled before working, to help strengthen them. If you wear an emerald ring, over time as you wash your hands the stone can dry out, chip, or crack.

It may also be surprising to see that quartz has only a rating of 7 too: If you drop a quartz crystal onto a hard surface it will break. Diamonds are the hardest of all minerals, well suited to being cut and shaped to bring out all their brilliance. Examples of minerals for each level of hardness are: 1: Talc; 2: Selenite; 3: Calcite; 4: Fluorite; 5: Apatite; 6: Moonstone; 7: Quartz; 8: Topaz; 9: Ruby; and 10: Diamond.

Mohs memorial plaque
This special plaque commemorates the work of Friedrich Mohs, creator of the hardness scale against which all gems and crystals are measured.

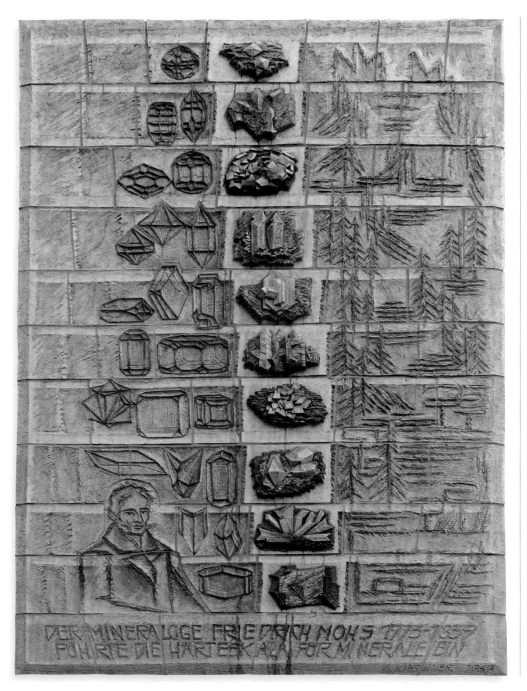

DER MINERALOGE FRIEDRICH MOHS 1773-1839
FÜHRTE DIE HÄRTESKALA FÜR MINERALE EIN

A. KIRCHNER 1957

Main Crystal Groups

Here you will see the main groups that crystals belong to according to geological classification. It is interesting to see how some of the crystals we have already mentioned fit into the geological ordering. The silicate group, which contains all kinds of quartz, plus feldspars such as moonstone or spodumenes such as kunzite, is the main group of stones associated with crystal healing.

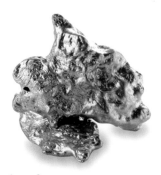

Native elements

These are minerals that occur in nature in uncombined or pure form. This category includes precious metals such as gold, silver, copper, or titanium, as well as other minerals such as lead, tin, nickel, or iron. Native elements occur as deposits in rock layers and are excavated all over the world; many are highly valuable minerals.

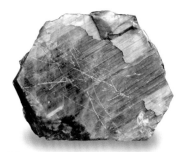

Oxides

Oxide group minerals form where oxygen combines with one or more metals present in the Earth's crust. For example, aluminum plus oxygen produces aluminum oxide, a compound also known as "corundum"; additional traces of chromium turn it red, to produce rubies, and additional traces of titanium and iron turn it blue, producing sapphires.

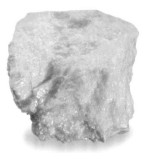

Sulfides

These mineral compounds contain the element sulfur, combined with a metal. For example, pyrite, or "fool's gold", is iron sulfide. Sulfide minerals are found either in veins, filling fractures, or cavities in rocks.

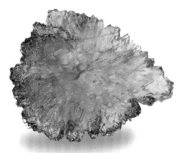

Mineraloids

These are mineral compounds which do not have crystalline structures. Many have a molten, glasslike appearance, for example, obsidian (volcanic glass), or tektites (meteorite glass, including moldavite).

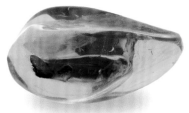

Organic minerals

"Organic" in the context of crystals means a mineral with plant or animal origins. Amber, for example, is the fossilized resin of an ancient pine tree. Pearls form when a grain of sand irritates the inner lining of the pearl oyster. Jet is a form of highly compressed coal.

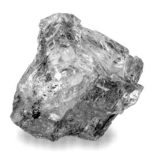

Silicates

The main category of minerals is silicon dioxide, making quartz, such as clear quartz, amethyst, rose quartz, smoky quartz, citrine, tourmalinated quartz, and rutilated quartz. In microcrystalline quartz, masses of tiny crystals appear in carnelian, agates, moss agate, and chalcedony; these stones have a more waxy luster. Also within this group are feldspars comprising a huge number of crystals that are common in the Earth's crust. Moonstone and labradorite are varieties of feldspar. Another large silicate group are garnets, which may be rich in aluminum, iron, or chromium depending on their location. Other silicate gemstones are tourmaline and the beryls, including aquamarine or emerald, as well as the spodumenes, including hiddenite.

CRYSTALS
THROUGH HISTORY

For thousands of years, human beings have been fascinated by gems. In early times, pieces of crystal were most likely found on the Earth's surface or discovered in caves. Used as symbols of power for ornament or in sacred ritual, these treasures of the Earth often held a special significance for our ancestors. In this chapter you will learn about the ancient heritage of crystals and their significance in major cultures of the world. You will also hear how crystals play a part in healing practices to this day.

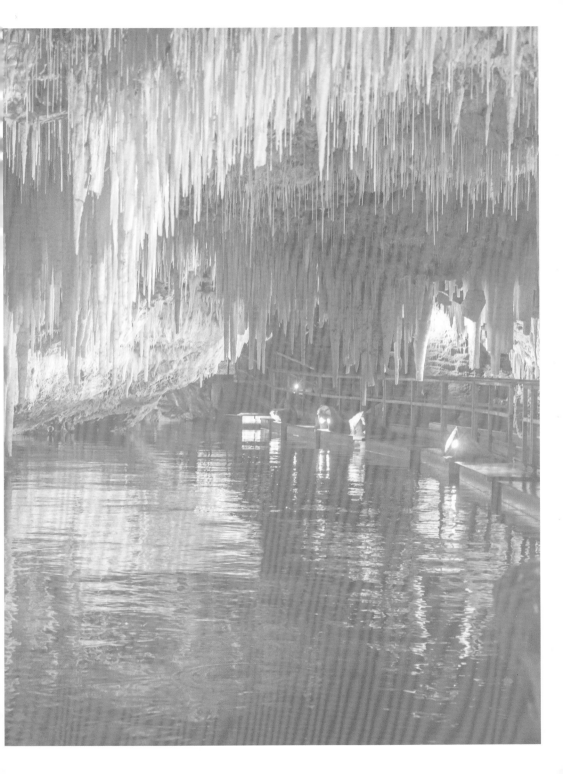

Crystals in Ancient History

Current archeological opinion says that as a species, human beings have walked the Earth for around 200,000 years. Most of that ancient history is totally unknown to us; the fossil record of the earliest humans is very sparse. We begin to pick up traces in ancient ancestral strains such as Neanderthal man, who became extinct around 40,000 years ago as a more modern species of human, *Homo sapiens*, began to increase in number.

Not just for decoration
The ancient tomb of Newgrange in Ireland is encased in quartz—used in crystal healing as a conductor. This gives the site a powerful energy.

Ancient archeology
Burial rites are a particular aspect of human behavior that sets us apart from other animals, and many archeological studies of ancient Neanderthal sites across Southern Europe have shown that Neanderthal people buried their dead with care. They often placed special objects around a deceased member of their family group, which may indicate that the objects themselves held a special significance. The remains of floral wreaths and collections of bear teeth, shells, and

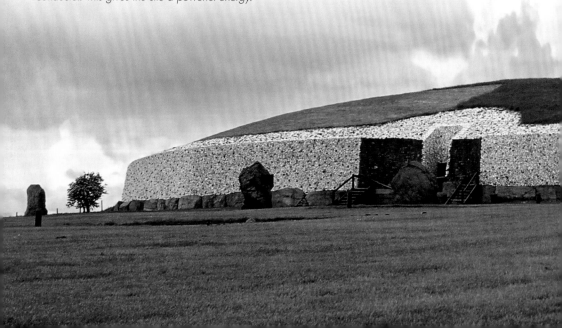

quartz crystals are examples of objects found in Neanderthal cave burials.

The way quartz sparkles when it catches the light would have made it easy to see among other rocks on the ground, and the way it sometimes shows rainbow patterns would have been intriguing. It is easy to imagine why these objects might have taken on a special significance to these ancient people. Of course we will never know precisely what the crystals meant to them, but their presence is still fascinating and suggestive.

Celtic history

Much closer to our time, the 5,000 year-old tomb mound at Newgrange in Ireland was finished with a layer of white quartz pebbles around the outer wall. This would have made the structure of the tomb shine out across the landscape. Other raised trackways and tombs from this era show a similar use of quartz. The reflective qualities of quartz clearly held a special significance to our forebears.

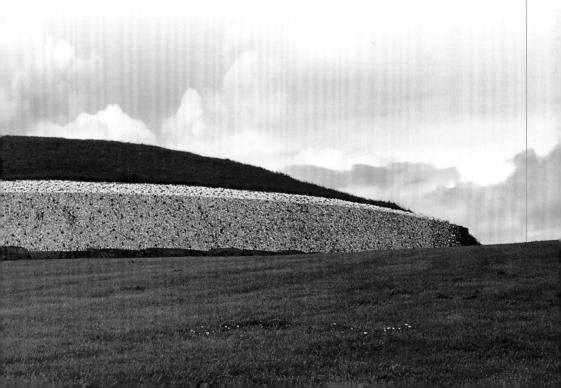

CRYSTALS IN ANCIENT CIVILIZATIONS

In recorded human history, great civilizations in different parts of the world have made extensive use of gemstones, crystals, and minerals as ornaments, precious objects, or ritual items. Countless examples of beautifully shaped and set crystals can be seen in museum collections all over the world, reflecting a passion that continues to this day.

India

The Indian subcontinent and the Himalayan mountain range have yielded vast treasures such as rubies, sapphires, and diamonds, as well as gold, silver, and copper metals, for at least 5,000 years. In Indian culture, ancient temple images and statues illustrate this clearly—bangles, nose pins, anklets, necklaces, rings, and more are shown being worn by both men and women. The wearing of gems and crystals was vital to Indian religious and ceremonial practice; in temples, statues of the gods were laden with exquisite necklaces as offerings from ancient Indian royalty. The energy of these beautiful stones was incorporated into a grand artistic tradition of human creativity.

Egypt

The wearing of crystals and precious stones as jewelry is found throughout ancient Egyptian history, going back as far as 7,000 years. Again, men and women wore all kinds of different adornments, including gold and silver items inlaid with precious stones. Higher-status individuals wore items with more complex designs, and the pharaohs, the kings and queens of ancient Egypt, had the most stunning examples of all. Most of the natural materials needed to make all this jewelry could be mined in Egypt or brought in from parts of Africa. However, one semiprecious stone was particularly significant to the ancient Egyptians: lapis lazuli, which comes all the way from Afghanistan. In the exquisite neck collar worn by Pharaoh Tutankhamun, lapis lazuli, jet, and carnelian were inlaid in gold. Crystals and precious stones were worn to show personal worth and rank, or as personal psychic protection from negative influences or harm.

The Maya of Central America

The ancient Mayan civilization was an extremely complex and advanced society,

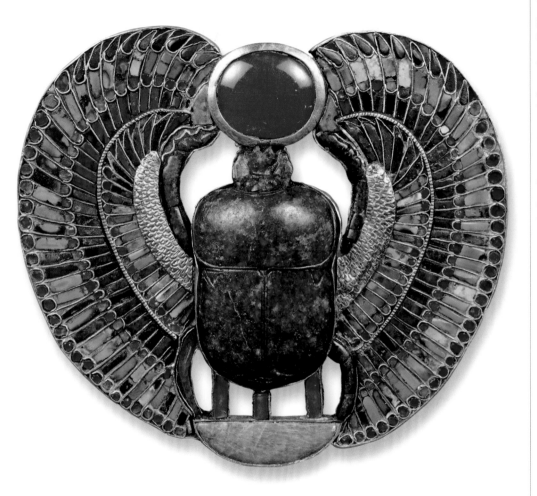

A tool for psychic protection

*This piece of Egyptian jewelry is called a pectoral
because it was worn over the chest. It was also an
amulet, designed to protect a person from evil
spirits. In a base of pure gold, it contains pieces of
dark-blue lapis lazuli, as well as pale-blue
turquoise, and orange-red carnelian stones.*

going back approximately 5,000 years. In Mayan society, the wearing of jewelry fashioned from gold and silver denoted status, particularly nose and lip plugs.

The Mayans were also miners of a type of jade called jadeite, a unique green semiprecious stone that they carved into jewelry such as headdresses, necklaces, bracelets, ear and nose plugs. Ornamental jadeite face masks carved from single pieces have been found in burial excavations, placed over the faces of ancient Mayan kings. The color green had a vital significance to the ancient Mayans, as it surrounded them in the jungles of Central America. Jadeite objects and ornaments were linked to the highest levels of ancient Mayan society.

China

Ancient Chinese cultures along the Yangtze river started to produce jewelry around 5,000 years ago. Like the Mayans, the Chinese venerated jade, which they carved into statues of dragons and other animals, as well as jewelry of many different kinds. Jade headdresses were worn by the Chinese royal family as symbols of status; jade was considered a talisman, capable of protecting the wearer from harm. Countless priceless

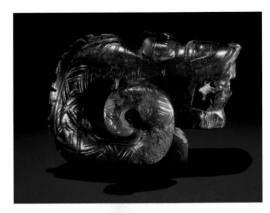

The beauty of jade
This carved dragon from China, ca. 1300 BCE, shows smooth curves and intricate lines that can only be achieved thanks to the softness of jade.

examples of jade carvings have been unearthed from ancient Chinese tombs, where they were buried with their owners.

The Chinese were also hugely skilled in metalworking of gold and silver. In 2011, a tomb was uncovered in Datong, a city in the Shanxi province of China, containing the body of a woman dated to 1,500 years ago. She was buried with astonishingly delicate yet elaborate earrings of pure gold fashioned like dragons, with two heavy amethyst teardrops that would have hung on either side of her face.

Mayan expertise
Skilled Mayan craftsmen worked with green jadeite to create complex pieces of ceremonial art, such as this funerary mask.

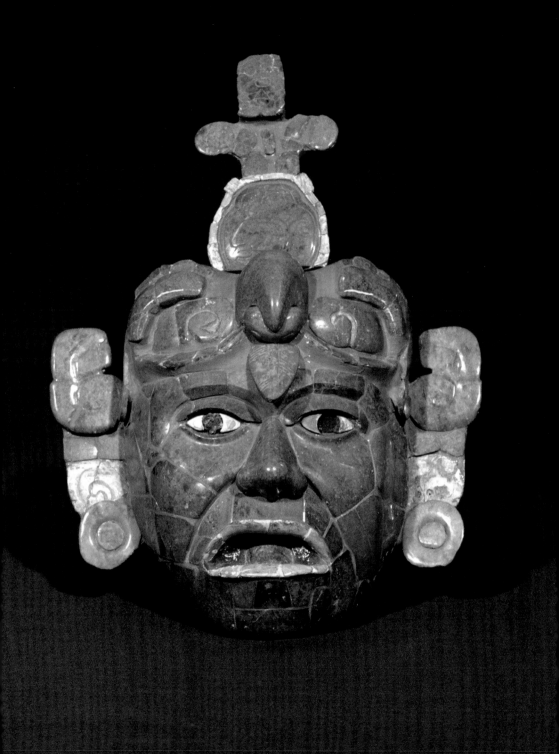

Crystal Healing in Modern Times

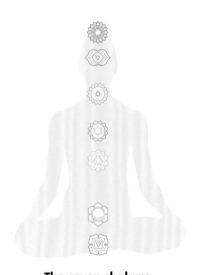

The seven chakras

This energy system underpins the practice of crystal healing.

As we have seen, crystals and precious stones have held a special significance for many different cultures at many different times. There are three main themes that emerge from the use of crystals in these cultures: first, the significance of wearing crystals on the person; second, using crystals to denote special status; and third, the use of crystals as ritual or protective objects.

Contemporary crystal healing

These three themes are still present in the practice of crystal healing, which developed in the latter part of the twentieth century as a holistic healing practice. This practice is based on beliefs regarding the energetic properties of crystals, according to their colors, shapes, and traditional uses. In crystal healing, stones are placed on or around the body of the person receiving treatment, so that they are surrounded by a matrix of crystal energy which protects and nurtures their aura, promoting personal healing and well-being. It may be suggested that a person wears a particular crystal that was used in their healing session to continue receiving the energy of that stone as they go through their everyday life. Guidance may also be given to buy and wear a certain stone because it is significant or special to that person, or to place one in their home for protection from negative thoughts or energy. In these ways, crystal healing practice still reflects the beliefs and practices of ancient cultures.

Complementary therapy

Crystal healing also links very strongly to different aspects of holistic healing such as color healing, in which the different colors of the rainbow are considered to have different physical, emotional, and spiritual effects: choosing crystals for their particular color plays an important part in healing practice. The seven energy centers of the human system, called the chakras, also benefit from the application of crystals to cleanse, balance, and restore energy. Crystal healing may combine crystals chosen for their colors and their links to different chakra energies (see pages 58–9).

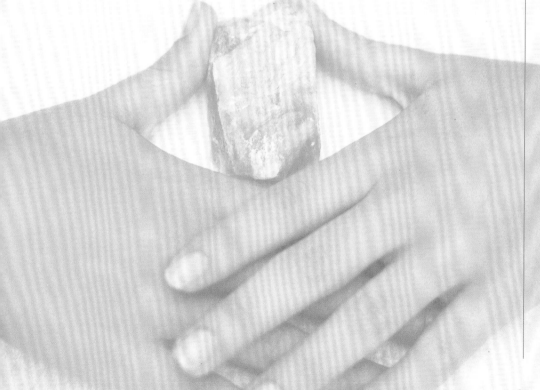

Crystals & Technology

Technical advances in manufacturing have led to modern crystals and stones that are either modified in some way or artificially produced. They are beautiful and work well as ornaments or jewelry, but in the practice of crystal healing, pure natural stones are always preferred because they carry energy from their original locations on or inside the Earth. Artificial or modified crystals are often sold alongside natural ones, so it is useful to be able to recognize them.

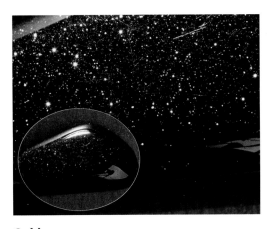

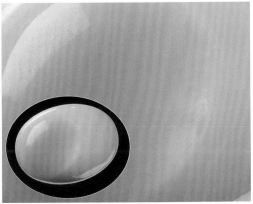

Goldstone

This is a type of glass in which tiny particles of copper are held in suspension as the glass cools from a molten state. The process for making it originated in Italy in the seventeenth century. Goldstone is either dark blue, showing up the copper particles like tiny glistening stars, or orange-red, with the same shimmer effect. It shapes easily and can be made into beads or pieces for jewelry, smoothed into tumblestones, or molded into figurines.

Opalite

This is actually a form of artificial glass made to show a milky effect with rainbow reflections. It resembles natural moonstone, though this crystal has a purer blue light reflection in it, or natural opal, which has a milky appearance and tiny fiery streaks of color. Natural opals are rare and very expensive, so opalite is often chosen for jewelry as an attractive and cheaper alternative.

Aura-type quartz crystals

These are pieces of natural quartz coated with metal atoms to create iridescent effects. Crystal healers have different opinions about aura crystals; some do not like to use artificially treated crystals, while others feel that the metals enhance the energetic properties of these stones. Examples of aura crystals include aqua, angel, and titanium aura quartz.

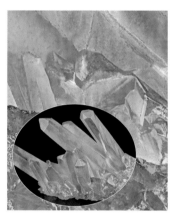

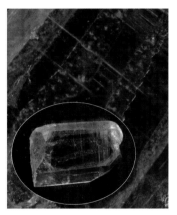

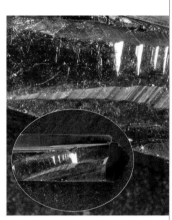

Aqua aura quartz

This is a form of treated crystal. Clear quartz is heated to extremely high temperatures, and fine gold particles are applied to the crystal so they fuse with the quartz crystal structure. When the crystal cools, it has a beautiful turquoise-blue shade with rainbow iridescence when the crystal is held at different angles. This form of treated quartz has become popular set in silver jewelry.

Angel aura quartz

The process for treating quartz to create angel aura quartz (also sometimes called rainbow aura quartz) is similar to aqua aura quartz, except that the super-heated quartz is bonded with particles of platinum and silver instead of gold. This creates a paler iridescence on all sides of the crystal without changing its basic color.

Titanium aura quartz

This is a form of treated quartz where the process of production is different. Particles of titanium are ionized onto the surface of the quartz; this is a cool process, which does not change or damage the structure of the quartz. Titanium is a conductor of electricity which makes this process possible. The end result has darker purple, gold, and turquoise-blue shades of iridescence.

BUYING & PREPARING CRYSTALS FOR USE

Find out how to start building your own collection of crystals, and how to look after them and prepare them for use. The more scrupulous you are when buying crystals, the better the energy they will hold; this makes them the best tools for healing purposes. As energy-absorbing and energy-holding objects, crystals need to be cleansed from time to time; this chapter discusses the best ways to keep your collection charged and refreshed, tuned to your energy, and ready to do healing work.

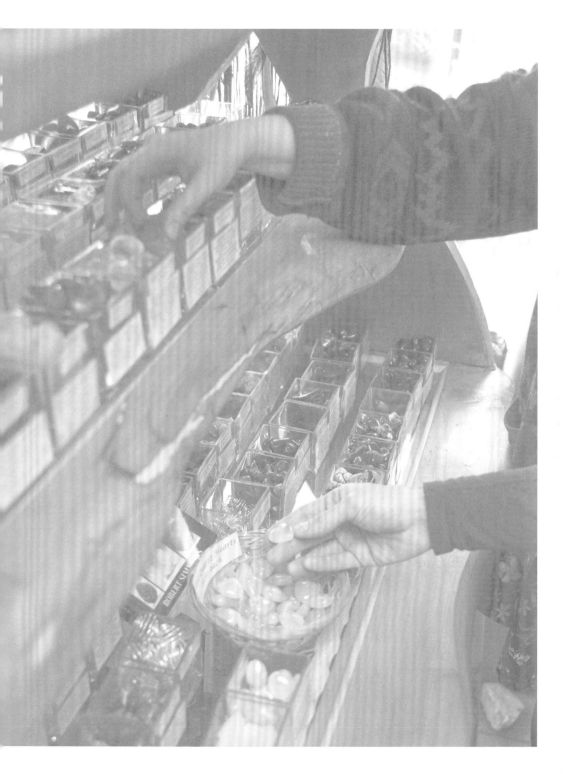

Selecting Crystals

Starting a crystal collection is a very personal journey in which your choice influences the kind of stones you bring together in a group. It is a reflection of your preferences and interests and also your energy levels—for example, if you find yourself buying several pieces of the same crystal at a particular time, then that crystal is "talking" to you, and you need its particular energetic properties. There are different ways and reasons to choose crystals; here are some examples.

Using your intuition

This is the most common way to choose a crystal: it "feels right." You can look at several pieces of the same crystal and one will "jump" out at you. This is purely an individual reaction because you sense something about the shape, color, or feel of a crystal that is beneficial and comfortable for you. As you buy more, you will find your intuition becomes more practiced; you will sense how some crystals feel more powerful than others. It is up to you to decide if a crystal with stronger energy belongs with you.

Choosing for color

Crystals appear in many beautiful shades, and this can be a big factor in choice. This chart shows some of the main crystal colors and their significance.

Color	Meaning	Common Examples
Clear	Clear and pure energy	Clear quartz
Pink	Unconditional love and gentle energy	Rose quartz
Purple	Expansive and spiritual energy	Amethyst
Blue	Cooling and calming energy	Blue lace agate
Green	Harmonizing and balancing energy	Aventurine
Yellow or gold	Revitalizing and brightening energy	Citrine
Orange or red	Warming and grounding energy	Red jasper
Brown, dark brown, black	Protective and shielding energy	Smoky quartz

Choosing for specific properties

While crystals are not a replacement for medical advice, many people choose them because of the properties they are considered to embody. On pages 66–7 there is a list of crystals showing their physical and emotional links, which you can use as a guide.

Choosing carefully

Holding two pieces of the same crystal will allow you to choose the right one for you, using your intuition and also looking at the exact shade of color.

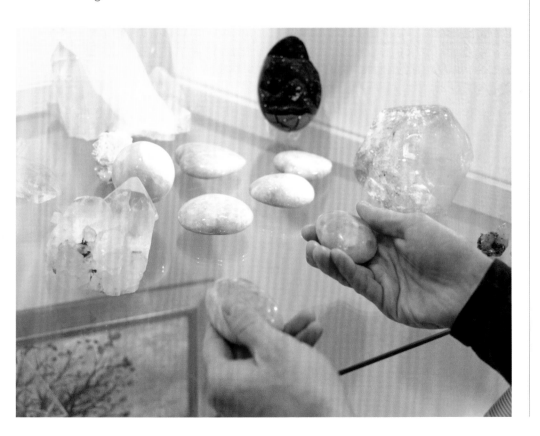

Choosing & Buying Crystals

Unless you are fortunate enough to have crystals given to you, or to find them amongst nature yourself, the likelihood is you will be buying them for your collection. In these days of internet shopping, a quick search will bring up countless crystal suppliers who sell all kinds of different sizes and shapes of stones. However, buying online is not the preferred way to buy crystals because you do not get to choose the actual stones you receive: the seller does that.

The best way to choose crystals is to see them, look at them closely, and sense which ones you feel drawn to. Do a search to see if there are any specialist crystal shops you can visit; it is worth going in person to give yourself the opportunity to be in that space with all the crystals and make your own careful decision. You may also find crystal fairs or special healing events in your locality where you can meet crystal sellers; again, these are worth investigation.

It is also good to sense how you feel about the person who is selling the crystals to you. To find out if the crystal has come from an ethical supply chain, talk to the supplier about where they source their stones, ask them if they know where they were originally from or if they know any of their healing properties. Reputable sellers take care to source from known contacts; however, as crystals pass through many hands on their way to the seller it can be difficult to track an exact supply chain each time. Buying from a caring and interested supplier means the crystals you end up with already carry good energy.

The right price

The wonderful thing about crystals is that there is something to suit every budget. Small pieces of crystal or round polished pebbles called "tumblestones" are very inexpensive and easily obtained. Medium-sized, more defined crystals such as natural quartz clusters are more expensive, and very large or rare pieces can be costly. If you are thinking of using crystals for healing, look for small to medium-sized crystals and use your intuition to sense which ones feel right to buy.

Get to know your local crystal store
Shopping for crystals is a fascinating and fun activity. Often you will find yourself spoiled for choice!

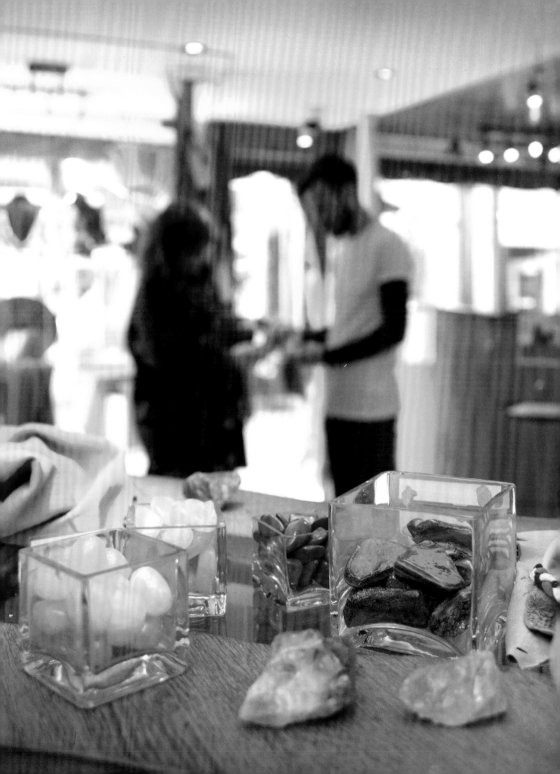

Cleansing Crystals

Crystals travel a long way before they get to you. They are extracted by mining in the countries where they originate, graded for shape and purity, sold on through wholesalers, and eventually reach the supplier you choose. By the time you buy them, they have been through many different hands, absorbing influences from each. It therefore makes sense to cleanse your new crystals to neutralize the energy they have encountered previously, making them ready to receive yours. As you keep your crystals, it is also good to cleanse them periodically to keep them energized.

Here are some ways to cleanse your crystals; choose whichever one feels right to you.

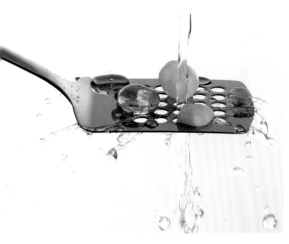

Water cleansing

A simple method is to hold crystals under cold running water, particularly when you first buy them. The water cleans away surface dust and old energy flows away, leaving the crystal sparkling. Afterward, pat them dry and place them on a soft cloth before you program them (see pages 46–7).

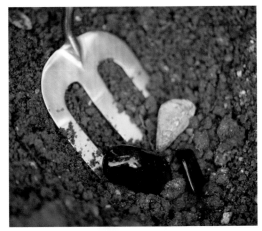

Earth cleansing

This method works best for protective crystals such as smoky quartz, black tourmaline, or obsidian, which absorb negativity. Every so often, bury your crystal in soil for a night: the Earth neutralizes any harmful energy it holds. Dig it up the next morning, rinse it under running water, pat it dry, and it is clear and ready to use again.

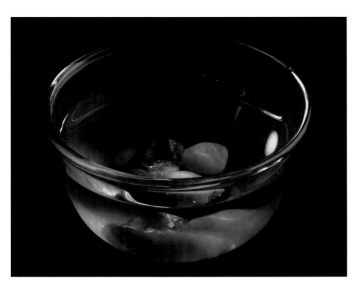

Moon cleansing

Use the gentle light of a full moon to cleanse your crystals, especially if you use them in healing. Place them in a glass bowl filled with mineral water, and leave it outside all night. The next day, remove the crystals, run them under flowing water, and then pat them dry.

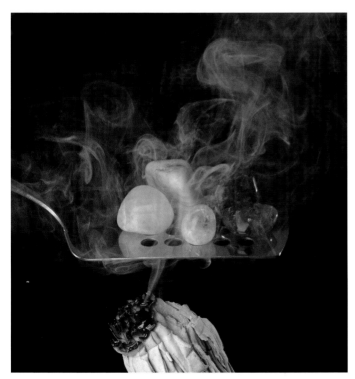

Smoke cleansing

Passing your crystals through scented smoke is called "smudging"; this also neutralizes any negative energy they may hold. You can use a scented incense stick; traditional Native American smudging uses a special kind of sage which you can buy as a "smudge stick" from New Age suppliers. Either way, you light the incense, and as the smoke rises, you pass your crystals through the smoke with the intention that they will serve the highest good.

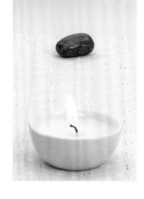

Create a quiet space
Before you start this activity, lighting a candle can help to create a peaceful atmosphere and heighten your focus

PROGRAMMING CRYSTALS
The idea of "programming" a crystal sounds like something out of computing, and actually the comparison is not so far-fetched. A program is a series of instructions a computer receives from a programmer that tells it what to do. The difference with a crystal is that you create the instructions and pass them to the crystal as you hold it and focus on it. The crystal absorbs your energy and the intention you create; it then continues to hold that energy pattern until you cleanse it and repeat the process again.

Programming crystals is needed when you first buy them and cleanse them; it brings them into your space, your energy field, and your life. Here is a simple ritual to help you do this:

Light a candle
After cleansing using one of the methods on the previous pages, prepare a space in your home—for example, a small table with a clean cloth on it. Light a small candle or tea light in a holder and place it on the surface, followed by the crystals you want to program. If you like, you can also light an incense stick. Sit on a chair or cross-legged on a pillow on the floor.

Be mindful
Sit quietly and observe the crystals you are bringing into your space. Breathe deeply and relax, feeling your feet in contact with the Earth, keeping your spine straight. Pick up a crystal and cup it in your hands, feeling its shape nestle there. Take a few deep breaths, then say out loud, "May you be filled with unconditional love and radiate into this space."

Bring variety
You can vary the instructions in your programming. Instead of unconditional love, for example, you can bring in

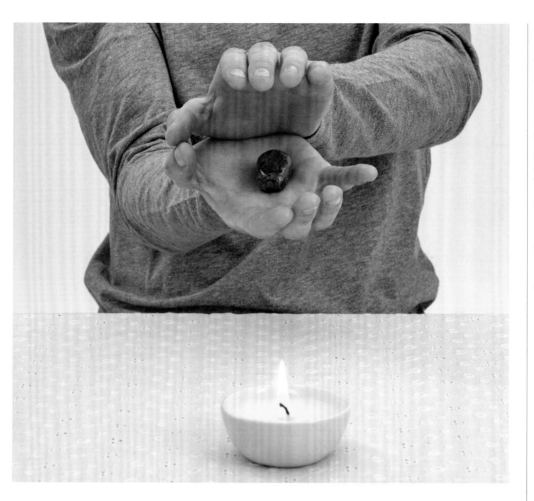

intentions for peace, protection, spiritual
growth, or healing, or you can program
a crystal to work with a particular energy
quality such as grounding, revitalizing,
communicating, earthing, expanding,
creative, or inspiring. You can also
change the program of a crystal any time
by cleansing it under running water and
repeating this exercise.

Focus your attention on the crystal

*Be aware of the shape, feel, temperature, and
color of the crystal as you hold it between your
hands. As you sense these qualities, you will feel a
connection to the crystal.*

47

Keeping Crystals

As we saw earlier on pages 22–3, crystals have different levels of hardness, and some are actually quite brittle. It is important to keep your crystals in ways that protect them from damage and maintain their beauty.

Preserving your crystals

Here are some simple guidelines:

- It is tempting to put your crystals on the windowsill to appreciate their color. This is fine for clear quartz, but naturally colored quartz such as amethyst can fade if left in sunlight.
- Be aware that most crystals will shatter if dropped onto a hard surface.

- Crystals with striations (visible vertical lines on their surface) such as selenite, or a very defined vertical structure such as kyanite, will tend to split along those lines if you drop or mishandle them. Be careful with them.
- Softer crystals such as amber will scratch easily, so avoid keeping them among any crystals with sharp edges.

The perfect place

It is also a good idea to think about where you keep your crystals. If you want to see them all the time, create a display in a corner of a room, preferably somewhere slightly out of the way so they will not fall

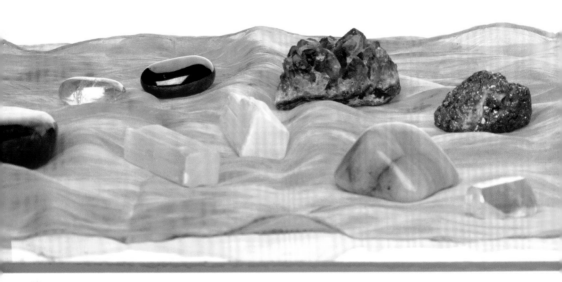

down and get damaged if people walk past. Crystals add beauty and energy to any room; some people like to incorporate them into an altar, to add a spiritual dimension to a living space.

If you want to see your crystals but you have small children who might be interested in them, putting them out of the way in a glass-fronted cabinet will still keep their energy visible.

When setting up a healing space such as a sanctuary for crystal healing work, placing crystals within that space is a lovely creative exercise. Perhaps you might decorate the space in colors similar to your crystals, so that when people come into the space they feel the color energies that your crystals radiate.

Should you want to take crystals with you when you travel, always wrap them up individually and put them in a special bag to protect them.

Create a display
Spreading your crystals onto a beautiful cloth is a simple way to display the shapes and colors of your collection, or to prepare a selection of crystals for a healing layout

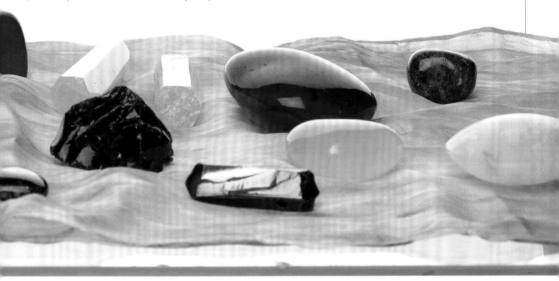

HOW TO USE CRYSTALS FOR HEALING

In this chapter, you will start using crystals to help yourself or your friends and family. Discover simple ways to feel the benefits of crystal energies using healing methods that enhance and support your well-being. Crystals can bring a new dimension to your daily life beyond just looking at them sitting on a shelf. They are energy companions, adding beauty and color to your space; they are also gentle and nurturing tools to help yourself and the people around you to feel more connected to the Earth's energy and healing vibrations. As you understand more about how to use them for their benefits, they will become a greater part of your life.

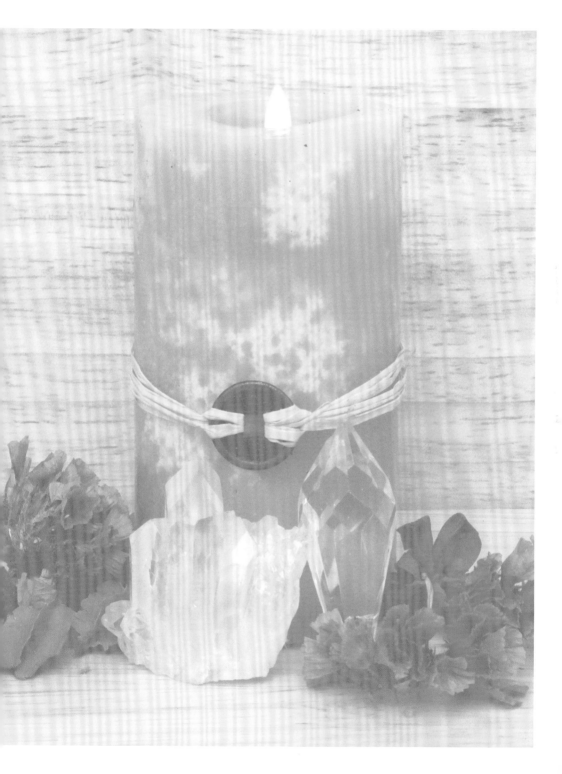

Meditation with Crystals

After buying, cleansing, and programming, there is another step to making a deeper connection with your new crystal. Meditating with it is a simple and gentle way to bring its energy closer to you, and to allow your intuition—your sixth sense—to share its vibration. It is a skill that improves with practice. If at first you do not seem to be sensing anything, do not give up; try a different crystal and see what happens. There are no rules here: it is all about your journey. You will find that you respond to particular crystals because your energy is more attuned to them.

Meditation exercise

This is a simple ritual to try for about fifteen minutes. Find a quiet place to sit comfortably, switch off cell phones and other devices, and ensure you will not be disturbed. Light a small candle or a tea light in a holder.

Choose a crystal for the exercise, perhaps a new one that you have cleansed and programmed, or a particular one that you feel is right for today.

Hold your crystal in your left hand and support it with your right hand cupping underneath. Take a few deep breaths and close your eyes.

Focus on the crystal. Sense its temperature, whether it feels cold, cool, or warm; feel its shape and texture, whether it is uneven or smooth and polished. After a few moments it will begin to take on the warmth of your hands. Then simply breathe gently, keep holding it, and experience what happens.

Sometimes you will feel a tingling in your hands as your energy is exchanged with the crystal; this may also be felt in different parts of your body. You may find that you begin to sense colors or see images of different scenes in your mind.

After about fifteen minutes, take a deep breath and open your eyes. Look at the crystal and compare how it seems now to how it did earlier. You may wish to make some notes about this crystal or draw any impressions that you felt or saw.

Pay attention to your posture
Sit on a firm chair with your back straight, your legs uncrossed, and your feet flat on the floor. This balanced position will help you to focus your mind.

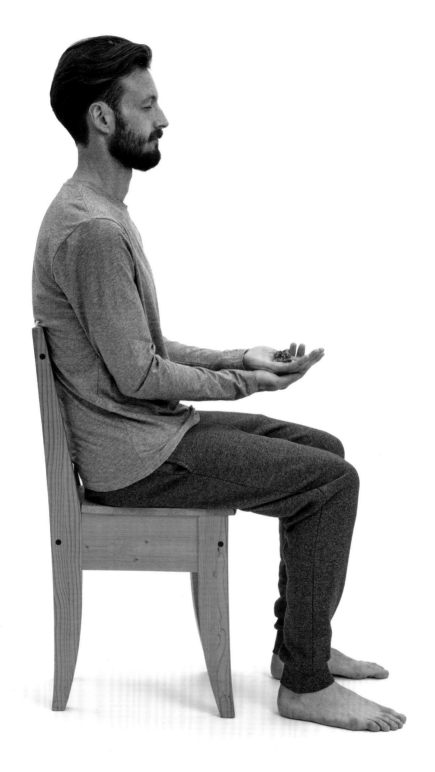

Wearing Crystal Jewelry

Many crystals and semiprecious stones are set in jewelry. Wearing jewelry is normally a fashion choice governed by the outfit you are wearing; however, with your new crystal awareness, you can also choose to wear certain kinds of stones for healing and protective reasons. It is a way of supporting your energy as you go about your day—and no one needs to know that you are doing this!

It is interesting to have a look at all the jewelry you currently own and see what types of stones you tend to wear. Understanding the properties and energies of these crystals may show you where you tend to need support. So, for example, if you keep wearing amber and you now know it symbolizes a need for physical energy, you might want to consider why your energy is depleted and perhaps do something about it.

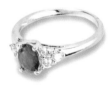

Silver settings
Wearing stones set in silver adds the properties of this metal, which is gently protective and soothing, reflecting the energy of the moon.

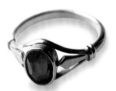

Gold settings
Stones set in gold are strengthening. Gold is energizing, powerful, and reflects the energy of the sun.

Carry the energy of crystals with you
Being aware of the properties of a crystal you are wearing can help you feel stronger and more centered throughout your day.

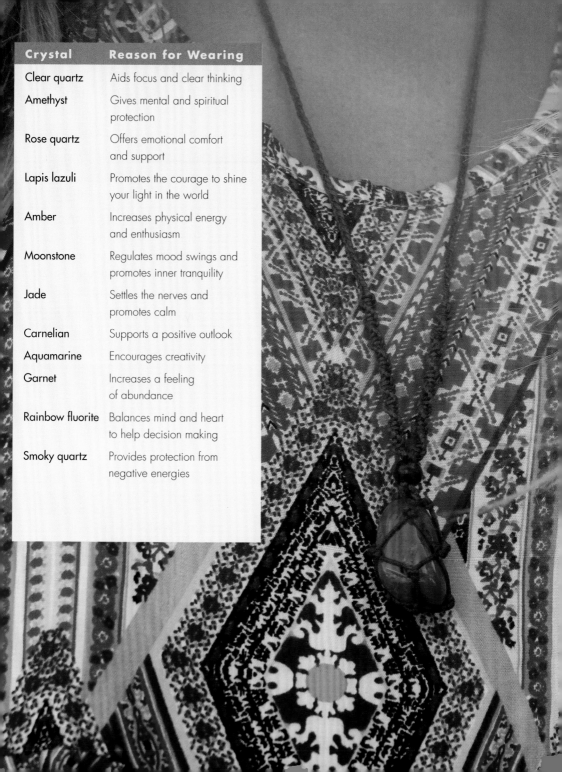

Crystal	Reason for Wearing
Clear quartz	Aids focus and clear thinking
Amethyst	Gives mental and spiritual protection
Rose quartz	Offers emotional comfort and support
Lapis lazuli	Promotes the courage to shine your light in the world
Amber	Increases physical energy and enthusiasm
Moonstone	Regulates mood swings and promotes inner tranquility
Jade	Settles the nerves and promotes calm
Carnelian	Supports a positive outlook
Aquamarine	Encourages creativity
Garnet	Increases a feeling of abundance
Rainbow fluorite	Balances mind and heart to help decision making
Smoky quartz	Provides protection from negative energies

Crystal Layouts: An Introduction

Making a crystal layout means placing crystals in a particular pattern to create an energy grid. This can be done by laying a variety of stones on a person or around their body; the combination in the layout creates a special field of vibrations due to the different crystals acting together.

Learning the art

Choosing crystals for layouts is an intuitive skill. It takes a long time to learn and experience the properties of many crystals and how they work best together: this is what crystal healers are trained in. However, there are simple layouts that can be tried as a beginner, with guidance as to where best to place crystals to feel their benefits.

When you are doing layouts, it is best to place a white sheet on the ground for the person to lie down on and a white pillow for their head. This creates a blank canvas to work on, and white is a color that reflects all the healing energy of the crystals being used.

Crystal mandalas

Another way of laying out crystals is to create mandalas—circular patterns of crystals laid on the ground. This can be done inside or outside to create a point of focus for a celebration, or to mark the full moon, or as a conscious act of Earth healing. Using a combination of crystals and natural stones can create beautiful patterns. Mandalas can be any size; sitting in the middle of a large pattern to meditate is a very energy-enhancing experience. Crystal mandalas are not permanent structures: they are placed as necessary and when their purpose is achieved, they are dismantled.

Intuitive mandala

To center your mandala, use a compass to align the cross with the four directions—north, south, east, and west. Any combination of crystals and natural stones can be used—your intuition will guide you to the best choice.

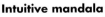

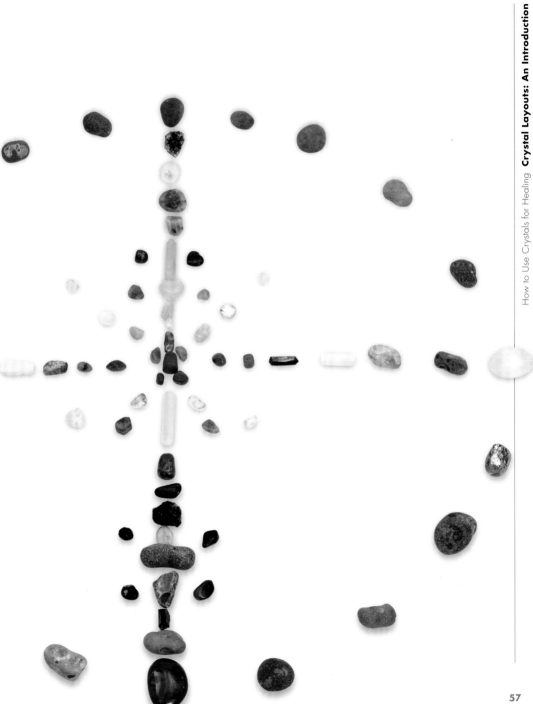

A SIMPLE CHAKRA BALANCING LAYOUT

This is a classic crystal healing layout that is used to balance the chakras, the seven energy centers along the spine. The seven chakras have different energetic vibrations and influence different levels of human life.

CROWN CHAKRA
This is the gateway to spiritual expansion; its colors are purple or white.

THIRD EYE CHAKRA
This is the place of intuition or the sixth sense; its color is dark blue.

THROAT CHAKRA
This is the communication center, mainly associated with speech; its color is pale blue.

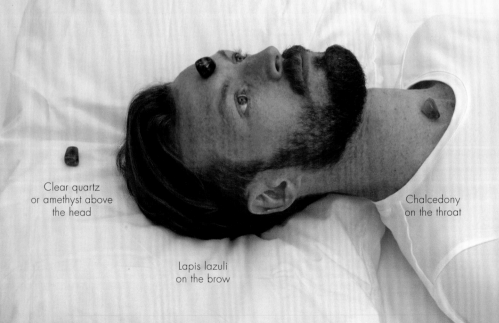

Clear quartz or amethyst above the head

Chalcedony on the throat

Lapis lazuli on the brow

In crystal healing, crystals in the colors of the seven chakras are laid on the body to stimulate and regenerate the energies of the chakra centers. The best kind of crystals to use for this layout are large polished tumblestones; a polished quartz or a small quartz point can be used for the Crown Chakra.

The subject should lie down on a white sheet with their head on a white pillow. Once the crystals are in place, they should then close their eyes and allow the energies of the crystals to do their balancing work. Rest in the layout for at least fifteen minutes to experience the benefits.

HEART CHAKRA
This is the center of unconditional love; its colors are green or pink.

SOLAR PLEXUS CHAKRA
This is the center of personal will and power; its color is golden yellow.

SACRAL CHAKRA
This is the center of sexual energy; its color is orange.

ROOT CHAKRA
This is the center that grounds and connects to Earth; its color is red.

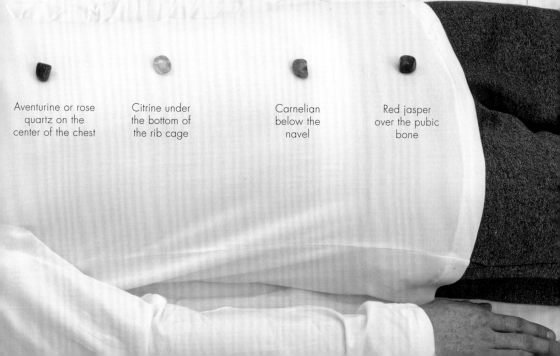

Aventurine or rose quartz on the center of the chest

Citrine under the bottom of the rib cage

Carnelian below the navel

Red jasper over the pubic bone

PROTECTIVE ENERGY LAYOUT

The aim of this crystal layout is to provide a protective space to screen a person from electromagnetic and environmental stress, allowing the body's energy field to regenerate and bringing a sense of inner peace and stability. We are surrounded by more electromagnetic stress than at any time during human evolution: from televisions, cell phones, tablets, laptops, radio waves, microwave energy, and more. We are bombarded with excess electromagnetic energy day and night; it even passes through walls. Conditions like insomnia, mental stress, and headaches are very common side effects of overexposure. Using this crystal matrix gives the body a rest from all this interference.

ABOVE THE HEAD
A selenite palm stone or small wand to cleanse the body's whole energy field.

ON THE BROW
An amethyst tumblestone to soothe and calm the mind.

OVER THE HEART
A bloodstone tumblestone for courage and protection from negativity.

ON THE SOLAR PLEXUS
A sunstone tumblestone for warmth and energy.

ON THE PUBIC BONE
A hematite tumblestone to give strength and connect to Earth.

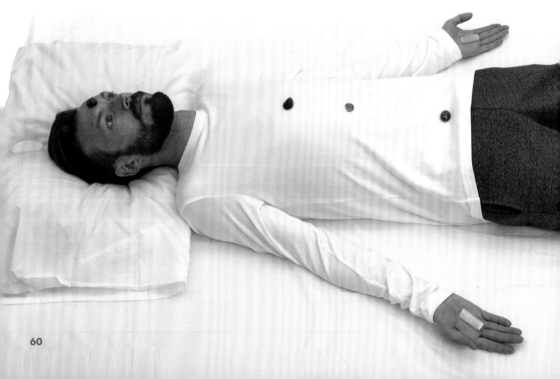

Protection While You Sleep

If you want to keep the energy of this layout working at night, you can place a selection of these crystals around your bed. Since it is hard to sleep with crystals lying on your body, you can instead place them on the floor, as near as you can to the level of the correct chakra, or create a "protective circle" by placing them intuitively around your bed.

BETWEEN THE KNEES
A smoky quartz for grounding and protection.

BETWEEN THE FEET
A snowflake obsidian to transmute negative energy into the Earth.

The subject can hold a small selenite wand in each hand for balance and to facilitate the passing of any negative energy out of the body's auric field.

Relax in this crystal layout for as long as feels comfortable. It is a beneficial combination to try in the evenings to feel deeply relaxed and at peace before you sleep.

HEART HEALING LAYOUT

This layout uses pink and green crystals to combine the two colors that symbolize the Heart Chakra's energy of unconditional love. Green is the color of growth, renewal, and life energy; pink is the color of gentle healing love. The image of a beautiful pink rose with green leaves sums up the Heart Chakra, and the crystals used here echo that pattern. This layout provides emotional healing for the heart; it is useful whenever a person is troubled, sad, or in need of comfort. It can also be used to regenerate the Heart Chakra at any time.

ABOVE THE HEAD
A medium-sized piece of rose quartz, either polished or tumbled.

ABOVE THE HEART
A piece of pink kunzite above the heart crystal to ease emotional stress and promote inner peace.

ON THE CHEST
A rose quartz heart in the center of the chest as a point of focus.

ON EITHER SIDE OF THE HEART
Two green aventurine stones and two pieces of chrysoprase to bring the Heart Chakra into balance.

BELOW THE HEART
A piece of green chrysocolla to clear any emotional toxicity.

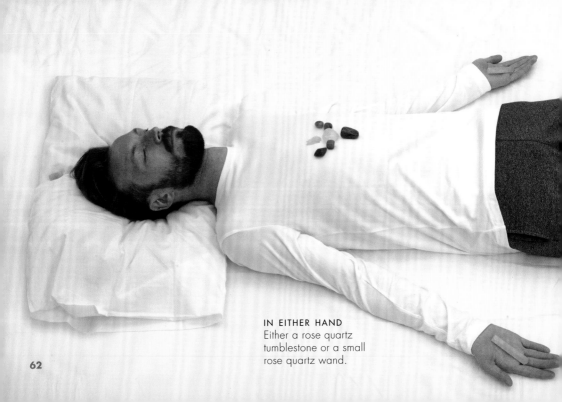

IN EITHER HAND
Either a rose quartz tumblestone or a small rose quartz wand.

Rest in this layout as long as feels comfortable, allowing the beautiful energies of the pink and green crystals to surround the body with their gentle healing light. Repeat this layout as often as needed to help a person whose heart is low and in need of gentle restoration.

BETWEEN THE FEET
A rose quartz sphere or a large rose quartz tumblestone.

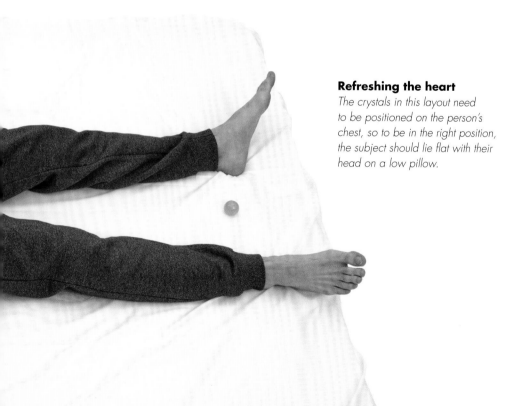

Refreshing the heart
The crystals in this layout need to be positioned on the person's chest, so to be in the right position, the subject should lie flat with their head on a low pillow.

Consulting a Professional Crystal Healer

Crystal healing is a holistic therapy that provides support and energy regeneration. Professional healers bring a detailed and deep knowledge and understanding of crystals and their properties to the sessions that they offer. If you are interested in exploring the effects of crystals on your physical, mental, and emotional well-being, it is worth consulting a trained therapist.

Crystal healers have different styles and approaches to their work, so it is worth speaking to a few and finding out more about them. Usually your instinct will tell you who feels best to work with. Ask them about their training, how long they have worked with crystals, and what kinds of treatment they offer.

The benefits of a healing session

These are some common themes for treatments:

- Removal of "stuck energy" patterns— old experiences that still cause problems, whether physical, emotional, or spiritual.
- Grounding and protective sessions to support people under stress.
- Balancing of the chakras in more depth, highlighting areas where energy is particularly out of harmony and working to restore it.
- Past-life regression sessions. These can be interesting to explore as a dimension of healing based on the idea of reincarnation.

Treatment will involve lying down on the floor or on a treatment couch with your shoes off, and removing any jewelry or watches as requested by the therapist. The chosen crystals for the session are laid on and around the body for the appropriate amount of time.

Multiple therapies

Many crystal healers are also proficient in other complementary therapies that work well with crystals, such as Reiki energy healing or color healing, which may form part of their treatment work. Crystal healing is a very individual experience and the therapist will adapt to the client's individual circumstances to help create a beneficial experience for them.

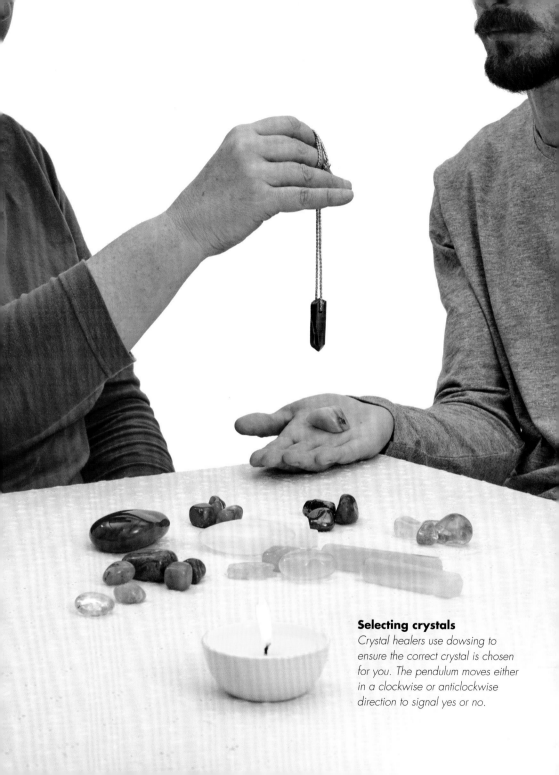

Selecting crystals

Crystal healers use dowsing to ensure the correct crystal is chosen for you. The pendulum moves either in a clockwise or anticlockwise direction to signal yes or no.

Crystals for Physical & Emotional Support

The following charts show crystals linked to different physical and emotional conditions. They are a useful source of guidance if you are looking for a crystal to support you during times of low physical or emotional energy.

Always consult a physician

Please remember that crystals are not a cure for these conditions. Holding them or carrying them is an added support, but for any serious issue you must obtain appropriate medical advice.

Physical Conditions	Recommended Crystals
Anemia	Bloodstone, hematite
Backache	Amber, danburite
Blood circulation	Bloodstone, ruby, hematite
Blood purification	Garnet, malachite
Cancer support	Rose quartz, watermelon tourmaline
Chronic fatigue syndrome	Ruby, amber
Detoxification	Smoky quartz, malachite, jet
Digestive problems	Green fluorite, amber, yellow jasper
Environmental pollution	Smoky quartz, obsidian
Headaches	Rose quartz, aquamarine, blue calcite
Hormone balancing	Blue moonstone, carnelian
Immune support	Malachite, rutilated clear quartz
Menopause support	Blue moonstone, carnelian
Menstrual support	Bloodstone, carnelian
Muscle aches	Hematite, red jasper
Skeletal support	Calcite (any color), fluorite
Surgical recovery support	Amber, rose quartz

Mental & Emotional Conditions	Recommended Crystals
Anger	Amazonite, rhodonite, lapis lazuli
Anxiety	Rose quartz, aventurine, amethyst
Assertiveness (to encourage)	Citrine, sodalite
Burnout	Carnelian, garnet
Communication issues	Turquoise, chalcedony, chrysocolla
Confidence (lack of)	Citrine, ruby, amber, red jasper
Courage (to build)	Bloodstone, hematite, carnelian
Creativity (to boost)	Iolite, lapis lazuli, apophyllite, charoite
Depression	Amethyst, angelite
Dreams (to calm)	Rose quartz, blue lace agate, black obsidian
Emotional distress	Lavender quartz, rhodochrosite, purple fluorite
Fear	Kyanite, aventurine, red jade
Focus (to build)	Fluorite (any color), pyrite, selenite
Forgiveness (to facilitate)	Kunzite, rose quartz
Grief	Self-healed quartz, rainbow obsidian
Grounding	Jet, smoky quartz, garnet, petrified wood
Insomnia	Amethyst, lavender quartz, smoky quartz
Irritability	Blue chalcedony
Jealousy	Citrine, prehnite
Joy (to increase)	Sunstone, citrine, amber, peridot
Love (to bring into life)	Ruby, rose quartz, peridot, chrysoprase
Meditation (to improve focus)	Lapis lazuli, iolite, celestite
Nervous tension	Aventurine, kunzite, watermelon tourmaline
Peace (to encourage)	Sugilite, seraphinite, brown jasper
Protection (to invoke)	Bloodstone, hematite, black tourmaline
Relaxation (to increase)	Rose quartz, blue lace agate
Self-esteem (to improve)	Amber, ruby
Visualization (to clarify)	Rutilated clear quartz, moldavite

Crystal Zodiac & Birthstone Charts

H ere are two other methods for classifying crystals, which can help you choose what to wear. One is the use of crystals as "birthstones"; wearing a stone associated with your birth month will have particular positive energy properties, especially if you wear it on and around your birthday. A second method of classification involves using your astrological birth sign; by wearing a crystal that symbolizes your sign, at any time of the year, you enhance the positive aspects of your sign in your daily life.

Birthstones

The accepted list of gemstones for each month of the year was defined by the National Association of Jewelers (now Jewelers of America) in the United States in 1912. Except for the recent additions of tanzanite in 2006 and spinel in 2016, the list has remained unchanged since then. Gemstones are the most expensive form of crystal, and this list encourages

the purchase of engagement rings set with a gem to match a person's birthday. The list of semiprecious alternatives is a selection of crystals with similar properties to the gems, but costing less to buy.

Month	Gemstone	Semiprecious Alternative
January	Garnet	Rose quartz
February	Amethyst	Onyx
March	Aquamarine	Bloodstone
April	Diamond	Clear quartz
May	Emerald	Chrysoprase
June	Pearl	Moonstone
July	Ruby	Carnelian
August	Peridot, spinel	Sardonyx
September	Sapphire	Lapis lazuli
October	Opal	Tourmaline
November	Topaz	Citrine
December	Blue zircon, tanzanite	Turquoise

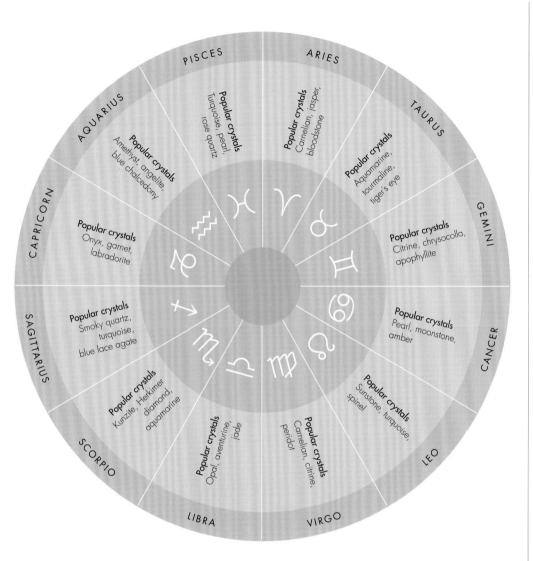

PISCES
Popular crystals
Turquoise, pearl,
rose quartz

ARIES
Popular crystals
Carnelian, jasper,
bloodstone

AQUARIUS
Popular crystals
Amethyst, angelite,
blue chalcedony

TAURUS
Popular crystals
Aquamarine,
tourmaline,
tiger's eye

CAPRICORN
Popular crystals
Onyx, garnet,
labradorite

GEMINI
Popular crystals
Citrine, chrysocolla,
apophyllite

SAGITTARIUS
Popular crystals
Smoky quartz,
turquoise,
blue lace agate

CANCER
Popular crystals
Pearl, moonstone,
amber

SCORPIO
Popular crystals
Kunzite, Herkimer
diamond,
aquamarine

LEO
Popular crystals
Sunstone, turquoise,
spinel

LIBRA
Popular crystals
Opal, aventurine,
jade

VIRGO
Popular crystals
Carnelian, citrine,
peridot

Zodiac crystals

It is also popular to list crystals according to the twelve zodiac signs in astrology. Match your star sign to the chart and see which crystals are indicated; you may find you have some of them already. Don't feel restricted by this list: if you like and feel drawn to other crystals that is fine. This is simply a fun way to link them to the zodiac.

Crystals & Feng Shui

Feng Shui, the ancient Chinese art of space clearing, healing, and placement, uses careful placing of crystals in your home to help balance the energy flow in your space. As a simple starting point, you need to know how your home sits in line with North, South, East, and West; check it with a compass and draw yourself a simple plan of your space to get used to its geography.

Feng Shui is an art in itself and this is only a very brief introduction, but here are some of the most popular crystals featured in this energy practice.

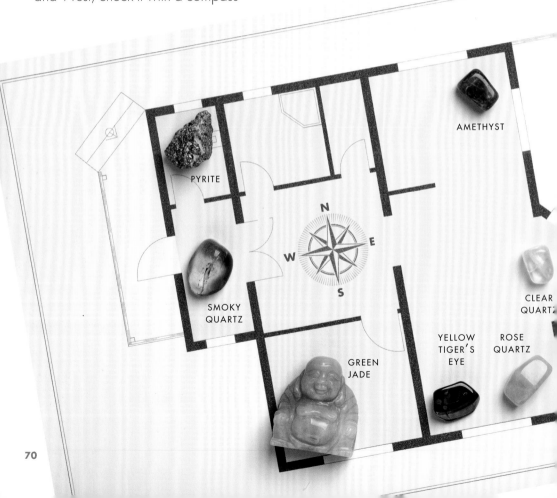

AMETHYST

PYRITE

N

W E

S

SMOKY QUARTZ

CLEAR QUARTZ

YELLOW TIGER'S EYE

ROSE QUARTZ

GREEN JADE

Crystal	Feng Shui Uses & Placement
Clear quartz	Clear quartz clusters are preferred in Feng Shui to cleanse and purify any space. Place a shining cluster in a prominent place in your living room to promote harmony.
Amethyst	The deepest purple amethyst crystals are preferred in Feng Shui. Locate the northeast area of your home—the place that promotes spiritual growth—to place a quality amethyst.
Rose quartz	Rose quartz works well in the southeast area of your home, symbolizing love and marriage. It also works well in children's rooms to promote sleep and peaceful energy.
Smoky quartz	Place a medium or large piece of smoky quartz by the front door of your home for grounding and protection.
Green jade	Green jade in the form of various types of carved figures are very popular in Feng Shui, particularly a Laughing Buddha placed in an office or work area for soothing and wise energy, or in the south area of your home.
Yellow tiger's eye	Yellow tiger's eye is used in Feng Shui as a focal point for strength and powerful earth energy. It works well on a windowsill in your front room.
Pyrite	In Feng Shui, gold-colored objects are used to attract wealth and prosperity and are usually placed in the northwest corner of your home. Pyrite's golden metallic sheen also brings energy to a work area or office.

CRYSTAL DIRECTORY

Explore the directory to find out interesting and useful information about ninety-four different crystals, their shapes, colors, and healing properties. You will find the clear quartz group of crystals featured first because this type is most commonly used in crystal healing. After this group, the remaining crystals are arranged into categories according to their use in supporting your well-being. Use the information in the directory to help you understand more about the crystals you add to your collection, how to use them for healing, and how to enjoy their presence in your life.

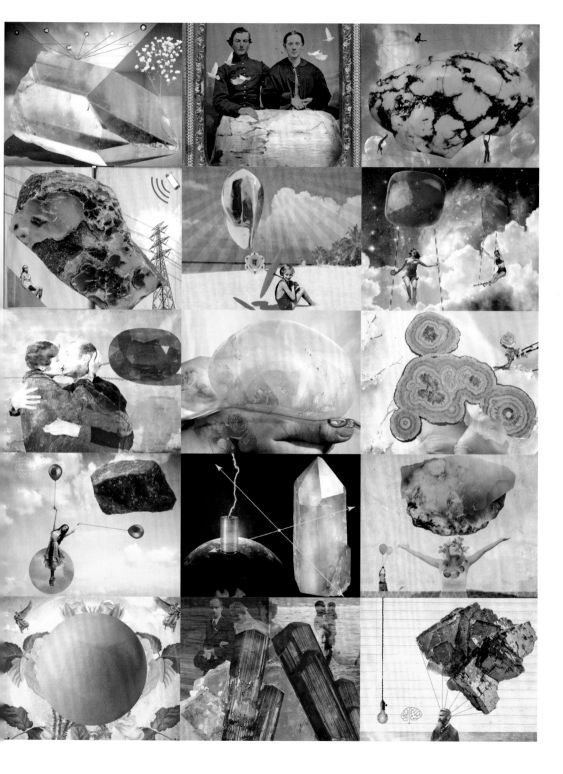

Clear Quartz

Crystal facts

Hardness
7

Color
**Transparent, with occasional
cloudy or white areas**

Geographical sources
**Mostly Brazil, US, or Madagascar,
but appears worldwide**

Rarity
Widely available

Form and structure
**Forms as six-sided crystals with
defined faceted points**

Chemical name
Silicon dioxide

To many people the word "quartz" is synonymous with "crystal," and this is not far wrong; it is probably the most commonly sold crystal in the world. The word "quartz" comes from the Ancient Greek word for "ice"; in the past, people thought it was ice that would not melt. Quartz is often found in granite rocks or alongside sandstone deposits. It appears in chunks, small points, or in large clusters in which points grow from a central core in diagonal directions; individual points have sharp geometric ends called terminations.

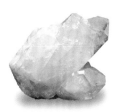

Most quartz is transparent, but some pieces contain milky or cloudy-looking areas. These effects are created by microscopic air bubbles trapped within the quartz structure. Sometimes entirely white pieces are sold as "snow quartz."

Quartz for well-being

If you are buying quartz specifically for healing purposes, look for clusters with very clear points, or for individual pieces with good transparency and clear six-sided end terminations. Quartz is an effective conductor of energy, and good-quality pieces are needed for healing work.

Clear quartz is one of the most versatile and useful crystals. It takes on the energy that is focused on it, so when you program a quartz crystal as we saw on

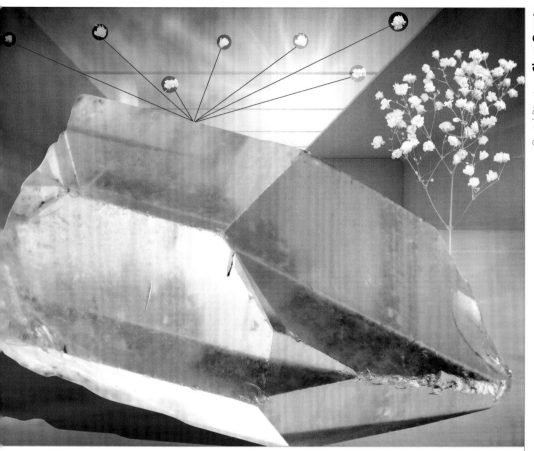

pages 46–7, this stone can hold and absorb that energy most efficiently. If you program your quartz to resonate with love, so it will do, and when you place it in a healing layout, it will continue to resonate that quality. Clear quartz is also a stone of light, reflecting and sparkling when placed in sun. It clears and cleanses a space, bringing a sense of brightness and ease.

Buying quartz

Clusters can be sold whole or divided into separate points. Small tumblestones are also available and can be polished up to a mirror-smooth finish. Prices vary depending on the size and complexity of pieces, but quartz is always affordable.

Clear quartz clusters and points can assemble in a variety of beautiful and unusual shapes. These unique variations have their own names, and in crystal healing have particular energetic properties. They are rarer and more expensive to buy than standard quartz stones, and make beautiful additions to a collection. On the next few pages you will see several examples of different types.

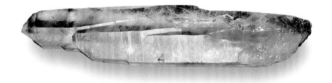

Laser wand quartz

These are long tapering pieces of quartz with finely sharp points. They have a bladelike appearance. As their appearance suggests, they have the ability to focus and transmit energy with laser-like precision; crystal healers use laser wands as psychic surgery tools, to remove particular energy blockages from the body or chakras with precision.

Directing the laser wand's point is like holding an energy scalpel in your hands. If you are drawn to this kind of quartz crystal it is useful to consult a crystal healer to learn more about how to use it for its beneficial effects; the use of it requires a very clear focus on what you are trying to achieve. This form of quartz is really for advanced crystal healing work.

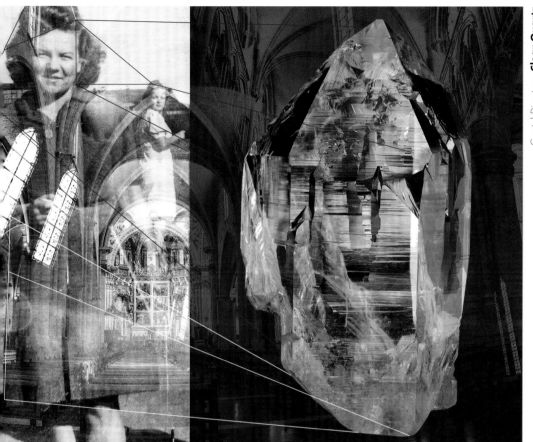

Cathedral quartz

This is a very beautiful and unusual formation in which the layers of quartz resemble the arching architecture of Gothic cathedrals. The geometric formation of this kind of quartz can lead to large pieces that have a unique presence when placed in a healing sanctuary. In crystal healing, cathedral quartz resonates with a body of ancient knowledge transmitted across time called the "akashic field." Holding or working with cathedral quartz amplifies your awareness of this ancient and mysterious field of knowledge to guide you in your healing work. Holding it in meditation may give flashes of awareness of past lives, or of other times when healing work was important to you.

If you are looking for the following unusual types of quartz, it is good to visit crystal healing fairs and talk to reputable suppliers. As we said on page 42, buying crystals online is not really advised because you cannot see or handle the stones before you receive them, and it is important that they feel right to you. When it comes to buying these more advanced forms of quartz, this becomes even more important because these are special healing tools.

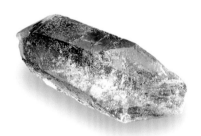

Self-healed quartz

This unusual form of quartz is usually double-terminated, that is, with points at either end. When looked at closely you will see that at some time the crystal has become damaged or broken, but over millions of years, new quartz has grown to cover and repair the irregular pattern of the break. This gives it the name "self-healed." This crystal is a rare form of quartz and it carries a very special healing vibration, which is great for using in crystal healing. Holding it assists people whose lives have been shattered by trauma, whether that may be physical, emotional, or mental. Self-healed quartz transmits to them the understanding that grief and trauma do pass, that self-healing is possible, and life experiences make us stronger.

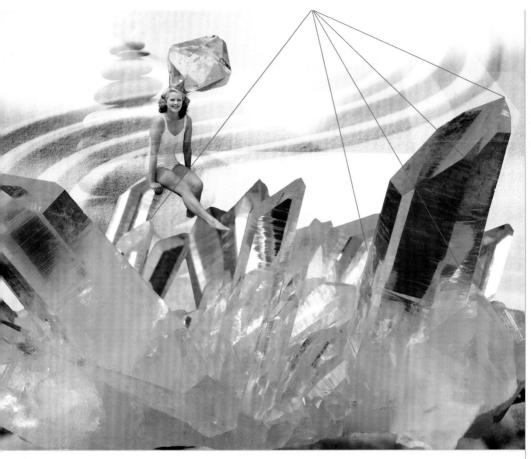

Abundance quartz

This quartz formation is made up of a cluster of small clear points angled in all directions, with just one or two larger points emerging out of it. The many angles of the crystal act as receivers and transmitters of light, and the larger points amplify the power of the piece. This kind of quartz brings in abundance in the form of light to be radiated into a space. This is a flow of energy that we need in life, not only to create money, but also well-being and positive energy for all. Place an abundance quartz in the northwest corner of your home—the abundance and prosperity area in Feng Shui—to draw more of these qualities into your life. You can also meditate with an abundance quartz crystal to receive its energy into your auric field.

The final two examples of quartz variations are
particularly rare and likely to be quite expensive
to buy, but they each have beautiful and unusual
formations and special energetic uses. If either of these
quartz formations call to you, it means that your energy
frequency is ready for them. If you are a beginner,
it is useful to talk to a crystal healer to learn more
about their particular properties and how to place
them for their best effects.

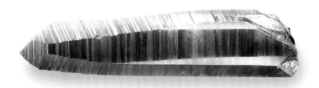

Lemurian seed quartz

This rare formation of quartz comes from
Brazil and Colombia. On the sides of the
long crystals you will see unusual
horizontal marks called "striations" at right
angles to the tip; you can feel them if you
run your fingers over the surface. This kind
of quartz often has a slight pinkish tinge.

It is called Lemurian seed because it is
considered to be linked to Lemuria, a
legendary continent that has disappeared,
where people had a deep and loving
connection to each other and the Earth.
Lemurian seed quartz symbolizes heart-
healing and the energy of love; it emits
a beautiful, gentle radiance that soothes
and restores the Heart Chakra center, in
the middle of the chest. It rebuilds and
strengthens feelings of Earth connection
and unconditional love.

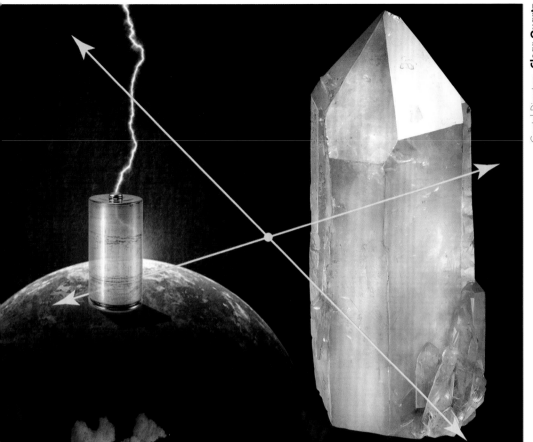

Generator quartz

This rare variant is a natural formation of quartz in which the pointed tip shows six perfect faces at exactly the same angle. This crystal has not been artificially cut and shaped: it formed like that itself. If you look at most quartz points you will see a variety of angles at the tip; absolutely equal six-sided natural formations are very unusual. These perfectly balanced specimens act like batteries that recharge the energy system of the body when it is extremely depleted or exhausted; they can be held or placed in a layout to help this process. A generator crystal can also amplify the energy of prayer or intention to send it out over a wider area. Placed on the Earth, they help to heal the planetary energy field.

Smoky Quartz

Crystal facts

Hardness
7

Color
Translucent shades of brown, from dark to light

Geographical sources
Brazil, US, Switzerland

Rarity
Widely available

Form and structure
Forms in large six-sided points or clusters

Chemical name
Silicon dioxide

Smoky quartz is another member of the quartz family and has a distinctive brown color, varying from light translucence to deep, dark shades. This quartz turned brown deep inside the earth in the presence of natural radioactive elements. It can be obtained in very large pieces, which have powerful energy, or as medium-sized chunks or small tumblestones. The color varies considerably, and you will be drawn to the shade that is right for you.

Since smoky quartz formed in the presence of radiation, the crystal "recognizes" different kinds of electromagnetic energy and neutralizes its effects. Its formation took place millions of years ago, so be reassured, these crystals are not radioactive! Smoky quartz will shield a person or a space from negative patterns. It is an excellent choice to place by your front door as a guardian for your home.

In the workplace

In an office, keeping a piece of smoky quartz on a desk helps to neutralize all the excess energy from laptops, tablets, and phones. Constantly sitting and working amid all this electromagnetic stress affects the human system, causing sleeplessness, mental strain, and insomnia. Smoky quartz works to keep your personal space shielded and clear. Carrying smoky

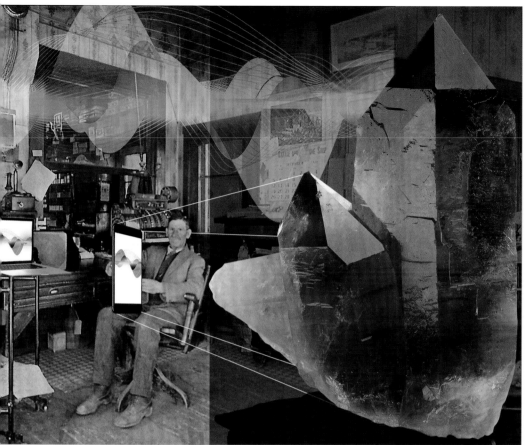

quartz with you as you travel to work and during your day helps to keep you grounded and focused; you will be less affected by the emotions and reactions of other people and able to keep your own energy centered.

Earthing yourself

In crystal healing, smoky quartz is used to create a strong, supportive energy field for the person receiving treatment, especially if their nerves are frayed by stress. Placing smoky quartz between the knees or below the feet helps a person feel grounded and safe. This is a crystal that helps to strengthen body and mind in times of severe stress or anxiety.

Turquoise

Crystal facts

Hardness
5–6

Color
Pale to deep turquoise blue

Geographical sources
**Afghanistan, US,
Australia, Middle East**

Rarity
Widely available

Form and structure
Forms as layered deposits

Chemical name
**Hydrated copper
aluminum sulfate**

Turquoise has been valued as a precious stone for thousands of years, and was worn as jewelry right across the world from ancient Egypt to China to the Middle East, to Europe and the indigenous peoples of North America. Its unique blue-green sheen comes from the blend of iron (green) and copper (blue) in the composition of the stone.

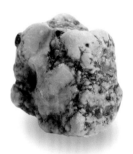

Turquoise has long been regarded as a stone of personal protection and good fortune. Carrying or wearing it attracts good energy and repels negativity. It opens perception to the realm of the sky, and hence to what Native Americans called the "sky beings," benevolent protectors of the Earth; you can invite their nurturing energy to guide your life. Turquoise symbolizes openness, freedom, and self-expression; it unites the green, expansive energy of the Heart Chakra with the blue, communicative energy of the Throat Chakra. In short, it encourages speaking one's truth from the heart. There is a popular saying that one should "walk one's talk." It means living and speaking from a place of inner personal truth. Turquoise is a powerful stone to wear to enhance your true energy and spirit.

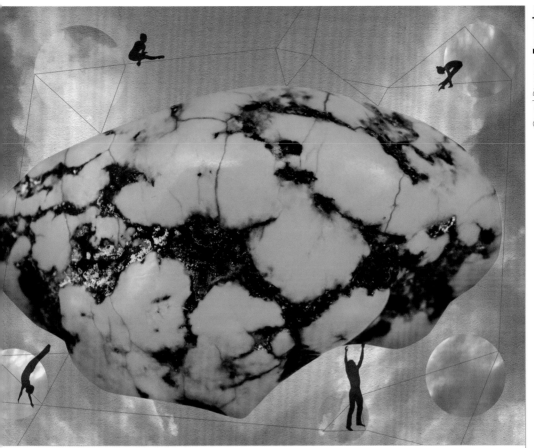

Crystal healing

In crystal layouts, turquoise can be placed over the Heart Chakra or the Throat Chakra to open and re-energize these energy locations. It helps people who cannot speak their truth, or who feel inhibited in their communication. Turquoise eases emotional stress and supports the renewal of positive feelings and energy in the auric field.

Color range

Different sources of turquoise from different parts of the world have varied colors; southern United States deposits tend to have a lighter duck-egg blue color while Middle Eastern deposits tend to be greener. Turquoise can also be mottled with white and black specks or have inclusions of gold pyrite.

Rutilated Quartz

Crystal facts

Hardness
7

Colors
Clear or brown with golden, hairlike inclusions of the mineral rutile (titanium oxide)

Geographical sources
Brazil, Madagascar

Rarity
Widely available

Form and structure
Forms as large, six-sided terminated crystals or as clusters

Chemical name
Silicon dioxide with rutile

Rutilated quartz occurs in two different forms: clear or smoky quartz, both with golden mineral streaks clearly visible within the stones. These are sometimes called "angel hair" because they look exactly like hair strands, but in fact they are strands of the mineral rutile within the quartz structure. Rutilated quartz has different uses and energetic properties depending on the type.

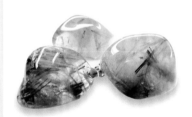

Clear rutilated quartz

Clear quartz with shimmering, golden rutile filaments is a crystal of transformation: it combines the clarity and energetic focus of the quartz with the conductive powers of the rutile. Holding it is like having a battery in your hands, where the energy passes even more quickly through the golden conductive threads. Clear rutilated quartz therefore moves energy swiftly through any situation and it clears negativity faster than ordinary clear quartz. In a healing layout, it amplifies awareness of higher forms of energy and is often placed above the head or on the forehead over the Third Eye Chakra, the psychic energy center. It is a good stone to meditate with if you are working to expand your spiritual and psychic awareness.

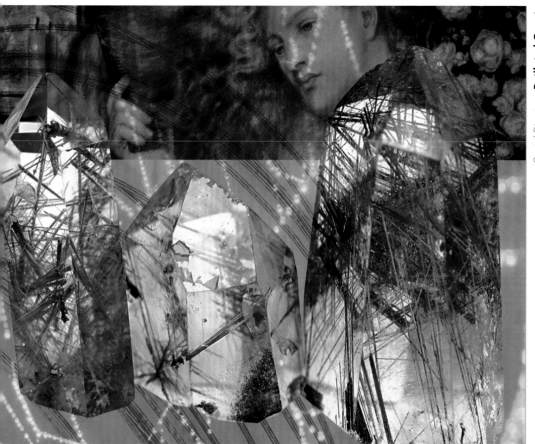

Smoky rutilated quartz

Smoky rutilated quartz acts as an even more efficient transformer of electromagnetic stress than regular smoky quartz. The rutile strands act as conductors to direct away negative energy straight into the Earth. Holding a rutilated smoky quartz and sweeping it around you in a clockwise circle is a wonderful way to clear and cleanse your space.

It is also a good crystal to carry with you to transmute any negativity during your day. It can strengthen your ability to let difficult energy pass into the Earth, so you remain grounded and positive.

Jet

Crystal facts

Hardness
3–4

Color
Black

Geographical sources
Britain, France, Poland, Russia, US

Rarity
Widely available

Form and structure
Forms when coal is squeezed between sedimentary rocks

Chemical name
Lignite

Jet is called a mineraloid because, rather than being a true mineral, it forms from plant fibers. Originally, waterlogged wood under layers of mud became compressed over millions of years to form coal; jet is a super-compressed, hard form of coal with a silky black sheen. It has been carved into beads, jewelry, and statues for centuries. Today it is available in raw chunks and polished spheres, tumblestones, or small carvings.

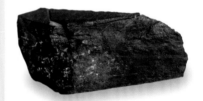

Jet's black color gives it protective energy; it has strong cloaking and shielding effects. Jet is similar to obsidian (see pages 204–5) and black tourmaline (see pages 198–9) in that all these crystals are used to clear negative influences from the auric field, grounding any negative influences into the Earth to be neutralized. Jet is seen as a gentler stone than the other two, with a more soothing effect, particularly on difficult emotions such as grief. It works well in healing layouts placed between or under the feet to anchor the body and allow blocked energy to be released. Placing a circle of small jet stones around a person lying on the floor acts as a grid, gently cleansing and purifying the entire auric field. Jet also has a detoxifying effect on the body, stimulating the kidneys to remove impurities.

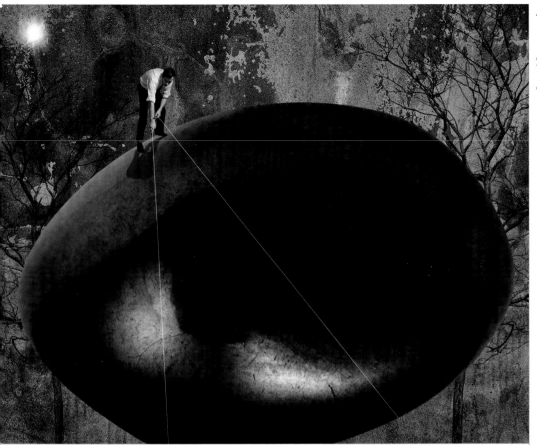

Making a safe place

Carry jet with you or wear it as jewelry during your day or when you travel; it shields you from negative energy, whether from people, places, or environmental stress. At the end of your day, particularly if it has been stressful, hold a piece of jet in each hand and meditate quietly to bring difficult emotions into balance and release them through your feet. Jet helps to give you a sense of strong support from the Earth, helping you to feel grounded and stable.

Moldavite

Crystal facts

Hardness
5–6

Color
Dark, leafy green

Geographical sources
Czech Republic

Rarity
**Rare and costly; source from
specialist crystal suppliers**

Form and structure
**Forms as amorphous
meteorite glass**

Chemical name
**Silicon dioxide with aluminum
dioxide and metal oxides**

Moldavite is a rare green meteorite glass from south-eastern Europe, and is named for the region where it is found. Moldavite belongs to a group of minerals called tektites, which are meteorite glass. Its formation is a mystery. One likely theory is that in the distant past, a large meteor crash-landed and split into many fragments. These white-hot pieces literally created a "splash field," scattering and melting the ground where they fell, forming greenish pieces of irregular-shaped meteorite glass in a radiating pattern around the impact area.

Moldavite came from a meteor that fell from space to Earth, and was birthed in tremendously powerful energy, powerful enough to vaporize and melt rock. It is not surprising, therefore, that the metaphysical meaning of moldavite is very powerful. It has been carried since ancient times as a protective talisman. Moldavite is also a crystal that symbolizes transformation from one state to another and the release of personal power. It releases energy in the body as a sensation of heat; some people experience this quite strongly when they hold a piece.

A powerful force

In crystal healing, moldavite is used to cleanse and re-energize the entire chakra system of seven centers along the spine. It can be placed on any of the centers to

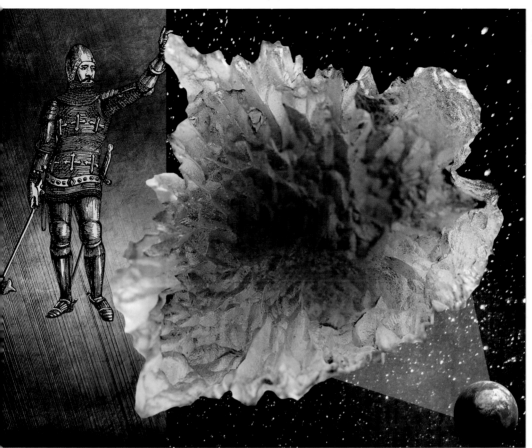

release blocked energy and restore
the flow through the spinal channel.
The power of moldavite is potent; its
transformative energy is supportive during
changing times or major life events. It
activates the entire auric field, so it is best
to experience its healing effects with the
guidance of a professional crystal healer.

Petrified Wood

Crystal facts

Hardness
7

Color
**Varied bands of brown
and black**

Geographical sources
**Greece, Australia, Czech
Republic, Argentina**

Rarity
Widely available

Form and structure
Forms as layered deposits

Chemical name
Silicon dioxide

Petrified wood is an unusual form of microcrystalline quartz. It formed over millions of years after trees fell in ancient bogs and were buried under mud layers which fossilized over time. The original cells in the wood were replaced by crystalline deposits of silicon dioxide; the shapes of tree rings can still be seen, but the trees themselves have turned into stone. Sometimes deposits of petrified wood are trunk-shaped and can be cut into slices big enough to make table surfaces for furniture. Mostly it is available as small polished pieces with varied patterns.

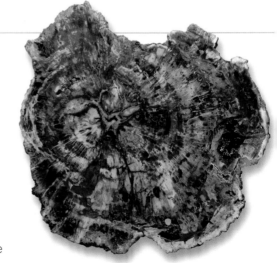

Petrified wood is a symbol of very slow change and evolution. It illustrates patience, and promotes the appreciation of steady growth rather than instant bursts of energy. Hence, it helps to slow down overactive impulses and bring a sense of quiet, calm acceptance that things will take the time they take. Holding a piece of petrified wood makes you think about the millions of years it has taken to change

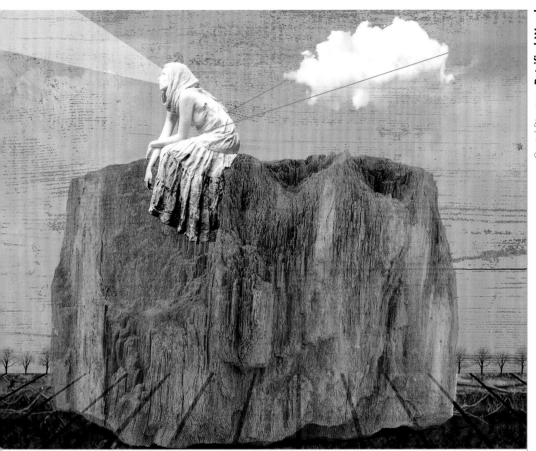

a tree into a stone; it gives you a sense of cycles of time that are vast, against which a human lifetime is only a blink. Many civilizations have the idea of the "Tree of Life" as a symbol: a great tree that sinks its roots deep into the Earth and has its crown in the sky. Meditating with petrified wood helps to connect to this Tree of Life, to the living organic presence of life on this planet through eons of time.

Strengthening your roots

In healing sessions, petrified wood can be used to calm and stabilize the Root Chakra, especially if the energy of the person being treated is very scattered or they are jumpy and nervous. Placed over the lower abdomen or on the base of the spine, petrified wood helps to anchor and stabilize the person's energy, bringing it back into a deeper Earth connection.

Onyx

Crystal facts

Hardness
7

Color
**Black striped with white
or gray; brown or white
forms also exist**

Geographical sources
Brazil, Germany, Mexico, US

Rarity
Widely available

Form and structure
Forms in layered deposits

Chemical name
Silicon dioxide

Onyx is a variety of microcrystalline quartz with a dense black appearance, sometimes with horizontal lighter bands running through it. Since ancient times it has been prized as a semiprecious stone, often carved into signet rings or seals to stamp documents. For centuries, darker-colored types of onyx have been stained to make them pure black, so be aware that pieces of a uniform color have been treated. For healing purposes, banded black onyx in its natural state is the best form to choose.

The white, gray, and black bands running through black onyx symbolize the interplay between the physical world and the unseen, or between matter and energy. Banded black onyx is a good stone to meditate with if you want to enhance your awareness of the magical realms. In particular, it helps you to remember that dark and light are simply different aspects of energy as a whole; in darkness, light is absorbed, and in light, energy is radiated. Black onyx helps you explore both, and stay balanced between them.

Maintaining harmony

In crystal healing, black onyx can be placed between or under the feet to stabilize the energy field during healing sessions. It can also be placed on the

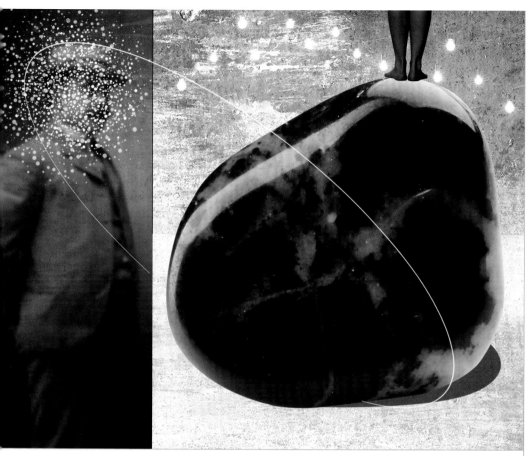

Root Chakra at the base of the spine to help anchor a person within their body. Keeping a balance between the spiritual and physical aspects of energy is important during guided healing sessions, especially when a person is seeking to expand their inner awareness. It is always good to stay grounded during healing work.

Malachite

Crystal facts

Hardness
3.5–4

Color
**Vivid emerald green with
distinctive bands**

Geographical sources
**Africa, Australia, Britain, France,
Mexico, Russia**

Rarity
Widely available

Form and structure
**Forms in massive deposits or
stalactite columns or in amorphous
"grapelike" structures**

Chemical name
Copper carbonate hydroxide

Malachite is a stunning, vivid green stone with beautiful paler green swirls running through its structure. When polished, it has a smooth and flowing appearance, and a silky surface. It can be found encrusted over other rocks, and is usually extracted during copper mining, as it forms alongside copper metal ore deposits. Due to its softness it can be ground into powder; like lapis lazuli (see pages 174–5), it is a mineral that the ancient Egyptians used as eye shadow. In ancient times it was regarded as a powerful talisman against negative energy.

Malachite continues to be used as a protective stone to this day. Its green, swirling energy acts like a cloak to the auric field. Carry it with you during the day or when you travel: it can shield you from unhealthy influences, including electromagnetic energy disturbances from computers and phones, and people who tend to leech your energy. Because malachite carries the conductive power of copper, it transmutes negativity and dissolves it. It is also a warrior stone; hold it or wear it when you need courage and strength to achieve your goal.

A healthy purpose
In crystal healing, malachite unites the Solar Plexus Chakra (personal will) with the Heart Chakra (compassion) so that personal power is used for the good of

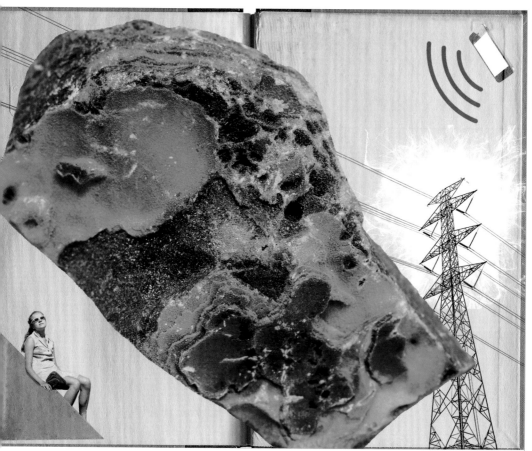

all. Placed over the Solar Plexus Chakra, malachite's conductive energy creates feedback with the Heart Chakra and clears the way for you to understand your higher purpose in life. Malachite is also used with other copper-based stones like chrysocolla (see pages 182–3) or turquoise (see pages 84–5) to stimulate the body's immune system and help recovery from periods of illness; these stones can be placed over the Heart Chakra and upper chest for a restorative effect.

Amber

Crystal facts

Hardness
2

Color
**Pale to deep golden yellow,
orange, red, brown, or green**

Geographical sources
Poland, Russia, South America

Rarity
**Widely available in the
golden-yellow form**

Forms and structure
**Forms an amorphous
(shapeless) structure as
pieces of fossilized tree resin**

Chemical name
Resin from *Pinus succinifera*

Amber has been collected since prehistoric times. To our ancestors, tear-shaped pieces of golden resin containing tiny pollen grains, seeds, or even insects must have seemed like magical objects. Amber is an organic material, not a mineral, as it formed in trees. Raw pieces are often opaque, but once they are polished their translucent golden beauty is revealed.

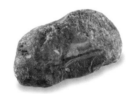

It took more than twenty-five million years for the resin from ancient Baltic pine trees (*Pinus succinifera*) to fossilize into what we know as amber. It is very lightweight and soft, so it scratches easily. Keep your pieces wrapped in soft cloth to preserve them.

Vibrant hues

Amber is usually golden yellow or orange in color, and this is the easiest type to obtain. Red amber is unusual and tends to be used in jewelry. Natural green amber is rare; most available green amber has been heat-treated or dyed. Because amber is so popular as jewelry it tends to be a crystal that is worn; however, raw pieces are sometimes available from specialist crystal suppliers. Golden amber links to the sun and its warming, radiant energy.

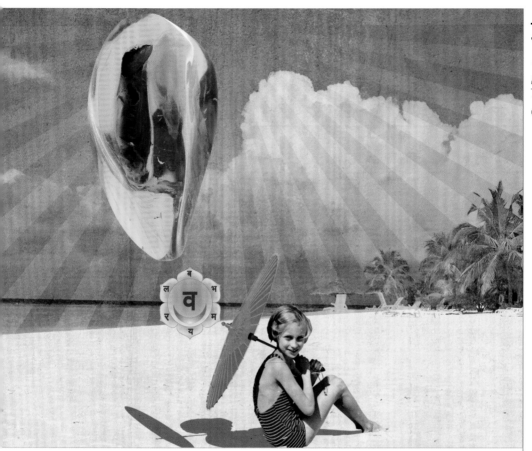

A sunny outlook

Wearing amber brings a sense of inner lightness and spontaneity, a feeling that all things are possible. Its sunny glow transmits positivity, optimism, and joy. Amber supports the energy of the Sacral Chakra (below the navel), assisting the digestive system, the adrenal glands, and the reproductive organs. It also helps to generate physical stamina and energy in the body. In crystal healing, raw pieces can be laid over the Sacral Chakra or the Solar Plexus Chakra (under the rib cage) to stimulate and regenerate these energy centers.

Bloodstone

Crystal facts

Hardness
7

Color
**Dark green with black and gray
mottling and specks of red**

Geographical sources
Australia, Brazil, China, India

Rarity
Widely available

Form and structure
Forms in large layered deposits

Chemical name
Silicon dioxide

Bloodstone is a colorful type of quartz in a group called chalcedony; in ancient times it was also known as heliotrope. It is silicon dioxide made up of tiny microscopic grains, colored green and black by different minerals present in the rocks where it solidified. The red specks in it are iron oxide; their blood-colored tint has given this crystal its traditional name of bloodstone. In ancient times this crystal was considered a powerful protector against physical harm and was worn or carried into battle as a talisman.

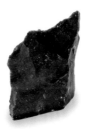

In crystal healing bloodstone is regarded as a "male" stone, but that does not mean it is limited to men. Rather, it means that it symbolizes masculine, outward-focused, "yang" energy that takes form in action. This kind of energy is needed by everyone to make progress in life and to generate positive change. Bloodstone is often placed over the Sacral Chakra (below the navel) or over the Root Chakra (over the pubic bone or on the base of the spine) to stimulate these two more physically-related energy centers. The energy of bloodstone can be balanced by placing "feminine" crystals with receptive "yin" energy over the Heart Chakra, such as rose quartz or pink kunzite. This combination of crystals harmonizes the masculine and feminine aspects of the energy field.

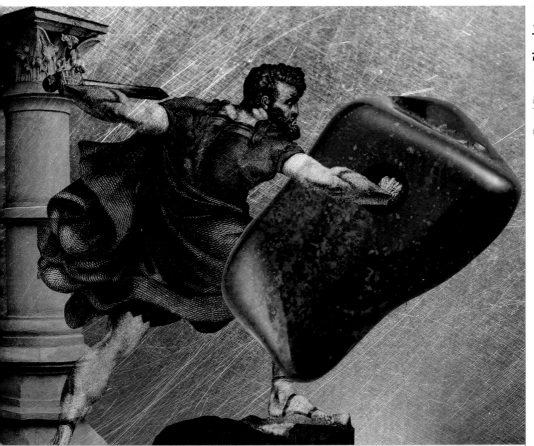

Finding strength

Bloodstone symbolizes courage, a spirit of adventure, and the ability to overcome obstacles. It is a good stone to carry on a journey to protect against negative people or situations. It also offers strong support at times when leadership is required, or simply when you have to "step up" for some reason and make your presence felt. Carrying bloodstone is like holding a shield to deflect any mental or physical blocks to progress. It gives a sense of steadiness and purpose.

Carnelian

Crystal facts

Hardness
7

Color
**Warm orange to deeper
orange-red**

Geographical sources
**Brazil, India, Iran,
Saudia Arabia, Uruguay**

Rarity
Widely available

Form and structure
Forms in layered deposits

Chemical name
Silicon dioxide

Carnelian is a type of microcrystalline chalcedony quartz. Tiny crystals form in banded layers colored by deposits of iron oxide, which turns the stone orange-red. The layers are squeezed into waves and lines by the pressure of surrounding rocks over millions of years. Carnelian can occur in opaque or semitransparent forms. It is often cut and shaped into spheres, smooth palm stones, or small, shiny tumblestones. It is very affordable and a common stone to include in a first crystal collection.

In ancient times carnelian was a stone carried to bring vitality, courage, and strength to the wearer. In crystal healing today, carnelian still holds that significance. It works with the three lower chakras: the Root (base of the spine), Sacral (below the navel), and Solar Plexus (under the rib cage). These three energy centers are a pyramid of physical, active energies, which are necessary to ground and center the spirit in the body. Pieces of carnelian placed over these areas of the body help to revitalize the chakras. People who need this treatment are generally those who are distracted, always bumping into things, or "in their heads." Carnelian is warming and grounding and balances body and mind.

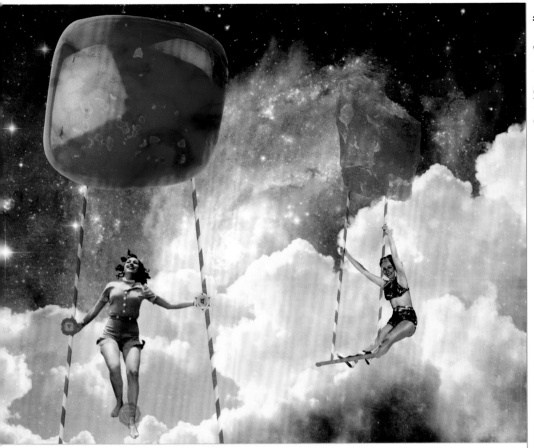

Living well

Carnelian also helps the body recover strength after a period of illness, such as influenza; holding the crystal or bathing with it helps the body absorb its supportive energy. This is a stone that warms the circulation and renews vitality. If you are nervous about staying true to your own purpose or feel unsure of your ability to do something, carnelian gives you the courage to act. It also encourages you to create and believe in your own destiny, roll up your sleeves, and get started.

Fulgurite

Crystal facts

Hardness
6.5

Color
White, beige, gray

Geographical sources
Africa, US

Rarity
**Rare; obtain from specialist
suppliers**

Form and structure
**Forms when sand fuses
into hollow mineral glass tubes
through lightning strikes**

Chemical name
Silica

Fulgurite is a special kind of mineral formation created when silica-rich sand melts in the presence of lightning strikes; this fuses the silica sand into glass, making long, irregular-shaped hollow forms. All fulgurite pieces are unique, and all of them have been created due to the violent interaction of lightning striking the Earth. Fulgurite formations are irregular, jagged, and twisted. They are mostly found in desert locations or on beaches after storms, and they tend to show the color of the sand where they originated.

Fulgurite is used in crystal healing as an extremely powerful energy channel. It has gone through metamorphosis—total transformation from one form to another. As when a caterpillar undergoes total metamorphosis into a butterfly, this transformation takes an enormous burst of energy. In these times of planetary instability when the news every day is of some disaster somewhere, fulgurite signals to us that we too have to change like this: humanity needs to evolve. For those who can accept the need for transformation, fulgurite is a powerful ally.

Respect the power
As fulgurite forms from a lightning strike, it makes sense that this crystal is an advanced energy tool and should only be used for healing purposes under guidance

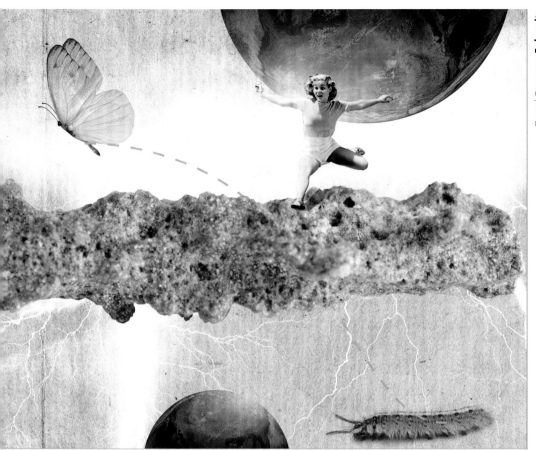

from a professional crystal healer.
Holding fulgurite can cause surges of very
powerful energy throughout the body,
and a crystal therapist can work with you
to make sure that your energy is supported
rather than overloaded. Fulgurite is not to
be feared, but it needs to be respected
for what it can achieve. For those who
are ready to serve the planetary purpose,
fulgurite is literally a "jump start."

Hematite

Crystal facts

Hardness
5–6

Color
**Metallic silver-gray
when polished**

Geographical sources
Australia, Brazil, Britain, Mexico

Rarity
Widely available

Form and structure
**Forms in massive deposits,
often in "grapelike" or rounded
structures**

Chemical name
Iron oxide

Hematite is an ore composed of iron oxide. When ground and mixed with water, the end result is blood-red, like the hemoglobin that colors blood; this gives the stone its name. Polished hematite has a smooth, silvery gray metallic sheen; it looks like a piece of molten metal when it is in fact a mineral. It is heavy compared to other crystals.

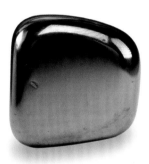

In ancient times, hematite was often carried as a talisman for strength and protection. In crystal healing today, hematite is used for similar reasons: it has grounding and strengthening energy, helping to dissolve anxiety and confusion. It works to support the Root Chakra at the base of the spine; placed there or over the lower abdomen in layouts, it helps to anchor spiritual energy into the body.

Hematite is a very good stone for people who are "too much in their heads" and who need to get back in touch with practical reality.

Feeling safe

Carry hematite with you during your day to give you strength and support in your work, and to protect your energy field from negativity. It is also a stone for

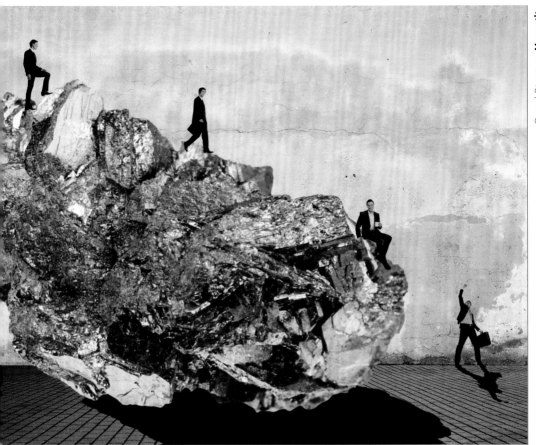

courage, for example, if you are going for a job interview or have an important task to do. The stone enhances your physical energy to help convert your ideas into actual results.

Hematite also stimulates the circulation, warming the body and preparing it for action. Meditate with hematite when you feel stuck or unable to make progress; feel its energy spread into your system, encouraging you to take that vital step forward. The message of hematite is: believe you can do it.

Peridot

Crystal facts

Hardness
6.5–7

Color
Golden green or olive green

Geographical sources
**Brazil, Myanmar, Pakistan,
Russia, Sri Lanka**

Rarity
**Widely available
(though mostly as jewelry)**

Form and structure
**Forms as small, short crystals
with a prismatic shape**

Chemical name
Magnesium iron silicate

Peridot crystals are small; another name for it is olivine, which refers to its beautiful green color. Peridot's particular shade arises from the presence of magnesium, iron, and small amounts of chromium and nickel. More than 3,000 years ago, the Egyptians mined for peridot on the island of Zabargad in the Red Sea; it is said that peridot stones were favorites of Queen Cleopatra. Today, peridot is sourced in many countries. Raw pieces are rare; most peridot is polished, cut, and shaped for jewelry.

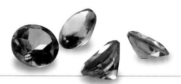

Wearing peridot brings a beautiful ray of golden-green light into your life. Peridot attracts love to you, so it is good to wear if you are looking for a partner. It is a crystal that encourages positivity, laughter, and joy; it feels good to wear it, especially if your energy is low and you need a boost. Peridot balances the Solar Plexus Chakra (yellow) with the Heart Chakra (green); it radiates solar brightness into the heart, opening it to new possibilities. Peridot also attracts abundance, so it is good to wear it and feel open to all the positive energy that wants to come into your life.

Fresh hopes
The spring-green shade of peridot also connects it to new growth in nature, to a sense of green vitality and lightness,

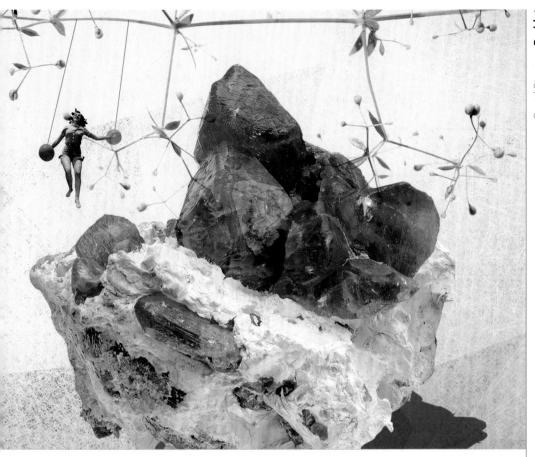

that positive feeling when the first green shoots appear at the end of winter. Wear peridot to encourage new beginnings in your life: when you see the signs, trust and follow your heart. It is a stone of good fortune and attracts auspicious results.

Pyrite

Crystal facts

Hardness
6–6.5

Color
Metallic gold

Geographical sources
Italy, Spain, Peru

Rarity
Widely available

Form and structure
Forms in cuboid or octahedral structures, often with striations (lines)

Chemical name
Iron sulfide

Pyrite also carries the name "fool's gold" because it has sometimes been mistaken for the precious metal. Actual gold, however, has a much more buttery yellow color, while pyrite has a paler golden sheen and a very obvious linear structure. It is often found with veins of quartz. Tiny specks of pyrite also appear in lapis lazuli (see pages 174–5). The name pyrite comes from the ancient Greek *pyr*, meaning fire; if you strike two pieces of pyrite together they make sparks. Pyrite can become brittle in damp conditions; make sure you keep it in a warm, dry place.

Pyrite's golden color connects it to the Solar Plexus Chakra, the place of personal power and will. It helps to energize you when you have tasks to complete; and is a good crystal to have on your desk where you work, to focus your mind and help you achieve your goals. Its angular structure helps to encourage discipline and logical thinking. Pyrite also has a bright, revitalizing effect on the entire body, increasing physical stamina and immunity. Carry pyrite with you to stay refreshed and energized during your day.

Vital energy
In crystal layouts, pyrite is either placed over the Solar Plexus Chakra or a piece is held in each hand to energize and brighten the auric field and detoxify any negative energy. It is sometimes called

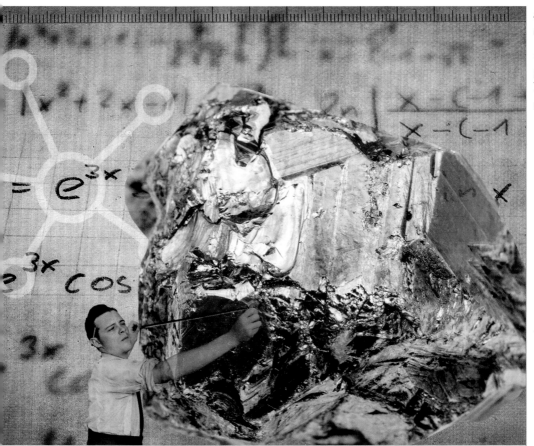

a "male" crystal, but actually its energies are necessary to both men and women: we all need to achieve things in life and find the energy to do what we need to do. Pyrite assists this process with a positive charge, giving a true helping hand. Placed with Citrine (see pages 136–7) over the Solar Plexus Chakra, pyrite helps to stimulate the flow of abundance into your life.

Ruby

Crystal facts

Hardness
9

Color
Crimson red as pure gem; lower grades are deep reddish-pink

Geographical sources
Afghanistan, India, Pakistan, Sri Lanka, Myanmar

Rarity
Gems are rare; raw pieces of lower grade are widely available

Form and structure
Forms as hexagonal crystals or prismatic shapes; also as granular deposits

Chemical name
Aluminum oxide

Ruby is one of the most precious of all gemstones, with a similar hardness to diamond. The finest-quality gems have a unique blood-red sheen which is even more dramatic when they are polished and faceted; this is due to chromium being present in the aluminum oxide. Some rubies have inclusions of titanium dioxide as well; these stones are cut and polished in rounded shapes called cabochons. The effect in the light is of a six-pointed star, so these are called "star rubies."

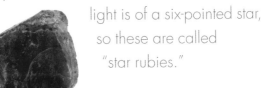

Ruby is a stone of self-confidence, of courage, and inner power. It encourages the belief that you can do whatever you dream you can do. If you are facing challenges, or some kind of test that pushes you beyond your comfort zone, then carry a piece of ruby as an ally, a support, and a reminder, saying "Yes, you can do this." Ruby stimulates the Root Chakra situated at the base of the spine, increasing physical strength in the body, warming blood flow, and providing you with the energy to act. Ruby is also a stone of passion; wear it or carry it with you to attract love into your life, or to ignite passion for the things that matter to you. If you are feeling low with no enthusiasm or energy for anything, then let ruby's deep red glow bring you back to life.

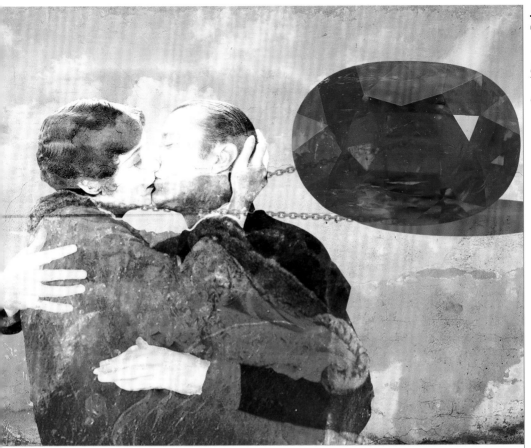

Revitalizing the heart

Gem-quality rubies are used in jewelry; however, lower-grade pieces of granular ruby are available and are used in crystal healing. In crystal layouts, ruby can be placed over the Root Chakra to stimulate and regenerate the body's physical vitality; it is good for people who always feel cold. Placed over the Heart Chakra, ruby warms the emotions and opens the heart to receive love. A piece can be held in each hand to regenerate and restore the whole body.

Sunstone

Crystal facts

Hardness
6–6.5

Color
Orange with sparkling inclusions

Geographical sources
India, Canada, US, Norway, Sweden

Rarity
Widely available

Form and structure
Forms in layered deposits

Chemical name
Sodium calcium aluminum silicate

Sunstone gets its name because, within its orange structure, there are tiny sparkling particles of iron oxide giving it an unusual sheen. Good-quality pieces have a high level of sparkle, lower-grade pieces less so. Sunstone has been sourced in Norway for hundreds of years and was especially valued by the ancient Norse people. Sunstone is available as small polished pieces or carved shapes like palm stones, eggs, or spheres.

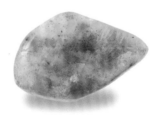

The bright orange color of sunstone always has a positive effect. It resonates with the Sacral Chakra just below the navel; its vibrancy revitalizes the body. It also encourages creativity and the drive that is needed to make ideas become real. Hence, this is an excellent stone to wear, carry, or place beside you in the workplace, to keep you feeling positive and self-confident. It also encourages you to receive abundance and let new things happen in your life. If you are going for a job interview or you have an important work meeting, then try carrying sunstone as an energizing source of support.

Brightening your life

In crystal healing, sunstone can be placed over the Sacral Chakra or the Solar Plexus Chakra to encourage creative energy

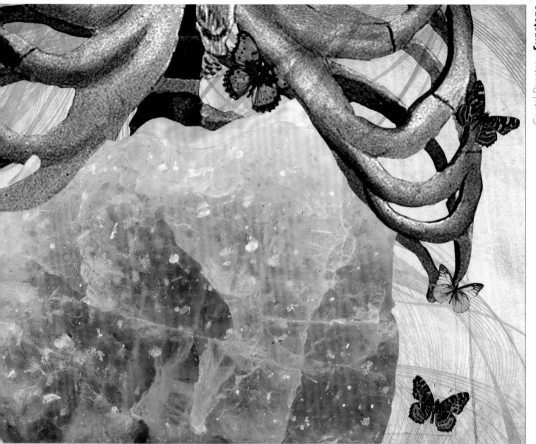

flow and a sensation of warm, bright energy in the center of the auric field. Sunstone helps anyone who feels stuck and unable to move forward, opening the mind to new paths and possibilities. It is also useful to revitalize the body and the auric field after a period of illness. Placed over the Throat Chakra, Sunstone encourages positive and joyful communication with others.

Rose Quartz

Crystal facts
Hardness
7
Color
Pale to deep rose pink
Geographical sources
Brazil, India, US, Madagascar
Rarity
Widely available
Form and structure
Forms in massive layered deposits, also in clusters or points
Chemical name
Silicon dioxide

Rose quartz is one of the most attractive and popular crystals available. It gets its color from tiny amounts of titanium and manganese that combine with silicon dioxide during the formation of the crystal. It often occurs in large masses with clearly visible cracks or faultlines in its structure; these mean it has to be cut and polished with skill. Rose quartz can be found in a clear crystalline form, but most often it is semitransparent or opaque.

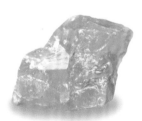

When choosing rose quartz for crystal healing purposes, look at both raw stones and polished pieces. Raw stones have their own particular qualities and color radiance; their irregular shapes are as nature presented them. Polished and shaped pieces, such as faceted wands, smooth spheres, and heart shapes, have been fashioned by human hands. Ask yourself which tool you prefer. There is no right or wrong answer here; it is what appeals to you.

The heart stone

In crystal healing, rose quartz symbolizes the heart, and it restores and regenerates the Heart Chakra in the center of the chest. Rose quartz radiates the energy of unconditional love, a healing ray of cosmic energy that supports and nourishes

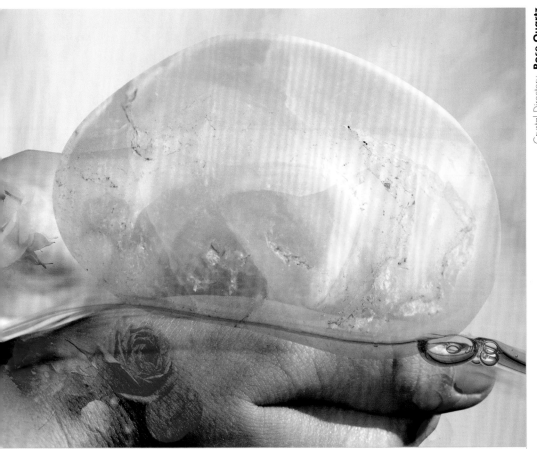

the whole human energy system. Holding it or placing it over the chest is the best way to feel its healing power. Rose quartz eases emotional pain and anxiety, and opens the heart to receive warmth and compassion. If you feel stressed, try taking a warm bath and putting a piece of rose quartz into the water; the crystal transmits its energy through the water into your body to soothe and calm you.

Lavender Quartz

Crystal facts

Hardness
7

Color
Pale lilac-pink

Geographical sources
Brazil

Rarity
**Rarer type of quartz,
more expensive**

Form and structure
**Forms in clusters or as
a large crystalline mass**

Chemical name
Silicon dioxide

Lavender quartz is another unusual type of quartz that has gained popularity in recent times, mostly because of its beautiful color. If you look at lavender quartz alongside rose quartz and pale amethyst, it becomes immediately obvious that the color of lavender quartz is a unique blend of pink and lilac, like a combination of rose quartz and amethyst.

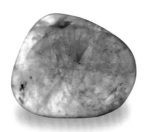

The name "lavender quartz" alludes to the pale lilac color of lavender flowers, and by extension this can be linked to lavender essential oil, in which the aroma of those flowers is captured as a pure essence of nature. Practicing meditation while holding a piece of lavender quartz and vaporizing or inhaling the scent of pure lavender essential oil, is an elegant way to experience the energetic vibration of this crystal. Like the effects of lavender essential oil, the energy of lavender quartz is gentle, soothing, and calming. It can ease mental and physical tension, and promote a sense of inner peace and tranquility. Meditating in the evening with this crystal and some lavender essential oil will help to ease insomnia and provide you with a truly restorative sleep.

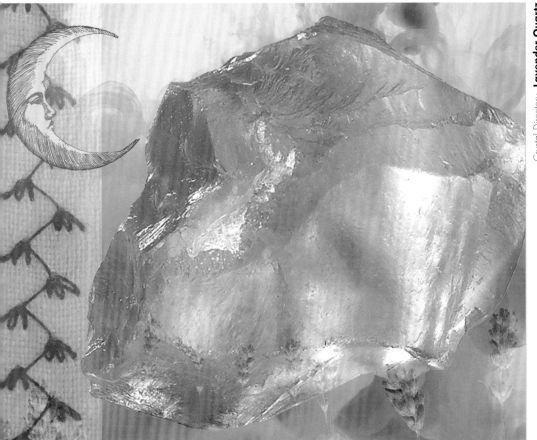

Nurturing colors

The two hues reflected in lavender quartz, pink and lilac, also have beautiful healing associations. Pink is the color of unconditional love, filling and nourishing the Heart Chakra. Lilac is a gentle ray of color, opening spiritual awareness. These two color rays combine to create the unique radiance of lavender quartz. Placed either over the Heart Chakra, or on the forehead over the Third Eye Chakra, lavender quartz nourishes the energy field with love and spiritual light. It is good for people who are experiencing emotional trauma or relationship difficulties, as it helps to balance heart and mind, easing the way to a clearer perspective.

Rhodochrosite

Crystal facts

Hardness
3.5–4

Color
Deep pink with white bands

Geographical sources
**Argentina, Peru, Canada,
South Africa, US**

Rarity
Widely available

Form and structure
**Forms as massive
deposits, sometimes in
rounded or stalactite shapes,
or as nodules within veins
or cavities in rocks**

Chemical name
Manganese carbonate

Rhodochrosite gets its name from *roz*, the Greek word for "pink"; its color is a deep rosy shade, and wavy creamy-white stripes run through its layers. Occasional specimens actually have crystallized deep-pink terminations (points), but these are rare. Large pieces of rhodochrosite are polished and made into spheres or statues; small polished pieces are easy to find. Every one has a unique pattern.

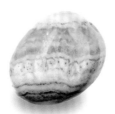

The rich rosy-pink color of rhodochrosite connects it to the Heart Chakra; it is a wonderfully supportive stone to carry in order to maintain emotional energy, especially at challenging times. It encourages trust in the heart, no matter what the outside world is saying. To feel the gentle, nurturing presence of rhodochrosite, focus on its deep pink ray of color by holding or placing a piece over your chest. Breathe deeply and let the crystal's rosy energy support you. Rhodochrosite supports people with delicate feelings, providing a cloak of loving pink energy. It also helps people to express their needs more easily, especially those who tend to be shy or introverted. Rhodochrosite is a good stone to carry when the heart needs courage to face new situations.

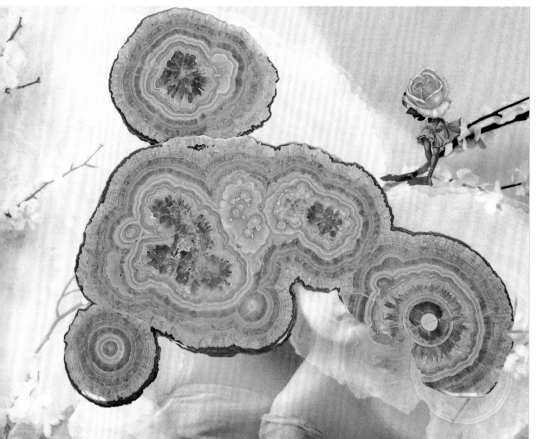

Creating comfort

Rhodochrosite can be used in healing layouts alongside rose quartz (see pages 116–7), pink calcite (see page 187), or kunzite (see pages 132–3) to create a pink energy grid on and all around a person. This kind of layout is very good for people who are feeling vulnerable, or who are grieving or in emotional distress. An alliance of all these crystals works well to support, protect, and restore the energy of the Heart Chakra.

Amazonite

Crystal facts

Hardness
6

Color
**Blue-green with paler
green specks**

Geographical sources
**Brazil, US, Russia, India,
Madagascar**

Rarity
Widely available

Form and structure
**Forms in large blocks or
chunks with defined angles**

Chemical name
Potassium aluminum silicate

Amazonite is a member of a large family of minerals called feldspars, which make up a significant proportion of the Earth's crust. As its name suggests, it is found in the Amazon region in Brazil. High-quality amazonite is also found in Colorado in the United States, and in parts of Russia. The blue-green color of the stone derives from a chemical reaction between lead and water as the mineral forms. When it is polished, amazonite has a smooth, silky feel; tumblestones or smooth palm stones of amazonite are comforting to hold.

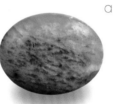

Amazonite's blue-green color harmonizes the energies of the Heart Chakra (green) in the center of the chest, and the Throat Chakra (blue) at the voicebox. It enables feelings and emotions to be expressed harmoniously and promotes loving and supportive communication. Hence it is useful to hold or carry in situations where there may be emotional conflict; the cooling, calming energy of amazonite helps to soothe inflamed feelings like anger or resentment.

Balancing head & heart

Meditating while holding or observing a piece of amazonite encourages spiritual communication between the heart and the mind, which helps with facing inner truths and the expression of one's true self. Holding a piece of amazonite and

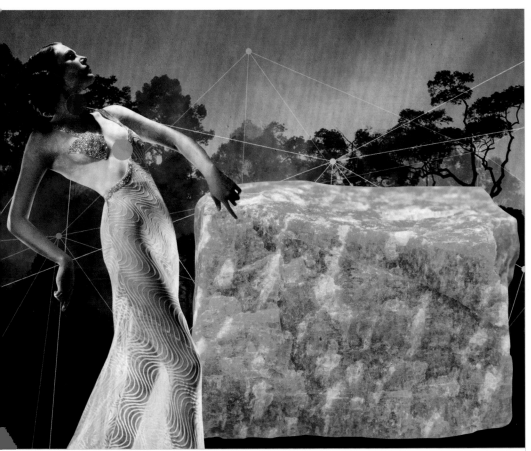

speaking your own healing intentions out loud amplifies the energy of your own spiritual purpose. This is a good practice at times when life is changing and your future path is emerging. Amazonite supports the feeling and expression of your new life.

In crystal healing, amazonite may be placed over the Heart Chakra or the Throat Chakra to encourage the balance of these two energy centers. It is often used alongside turquoise or chrysocolla (other blue-green stones) to enhance communication between the two chakras.

Aquamarine

Aquamarine is a member of the group of crystals called beryl, which also includes emeralds. These crystals are gemstones; the highest-quality pieces are cut, faceted, and fashioned into expensive jewelry such as rings or necklaces. For the crystal collector, lower-grade and slightly more opaque pieces of aquamarine are available; these still carry that lovely translucent pale turquoise color.

The name "aquamarine" literally means "sea water"; the color of the crystal reflects the color of the sea. This crystal links to the water element, to feelings and emotions, to tears, and to the waters of life. It is a cleansing crystal; its gentle energy bathes the heart and eases away emotional tension and heartache. It is very good to hold or meditate with aquamarine to let go of grief or deeply held feelings. Aquamarine also cools the body and eases overly inflamed emotions or physical inflammation.

Opening up

Aquamarine acts as a balance between the Throat Chakra (associated with the color blue) and Heart Chakra (associated with green) on a very gentle and spiritual level, promoting the calm expression of

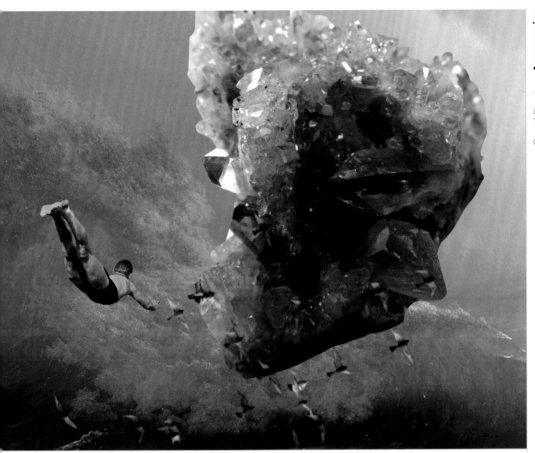

personal truth. It works well for anyone who has difficulty speaking about feelings; aquamarine opens the way to self-expression. It is also a good stone to carry if you have to speak in company, give a presentation, or perform in some way. Aquamarine enhances the energy of your communication.

Placing aquamarine over the Heart Chakra (center of chest) or the Throat Chakra area cools and soothes those energy centers. Placing a piece over the Third Eye Chakra (the psychic center in the middle of the forehead) can help you connect to the spiritual energy of the sea and its creatures, bringing a sense of expansion and freedom.

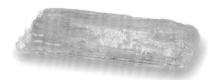

Aventurine

Crystal facts

Hardness
7

Color
Light to rich green with tiny lighter specks

Geographical sources
Brazil, India, Russia

Rarity
Widely available

Form and structure
Forms as microcrystalline quartz in large layered deposits

Chemical name
Silicon dioxide

Aventurine is a lovely green stone with touches of sparkling iridescence when you turn it to the light, thanks to particles of green chromium within its structure. It is a form of microcrystalline quartz, meaning it is made up of silicon dioxide in tiny microscopic granules, compressed by heat into layers within rocks. All types of microcrystalline quartz have a milky, semitransparent appearance when polished. Aventurine is classed as a semiprecious stone; quality pieces make beautiful jewelry.

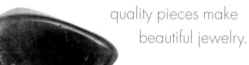

Aventurine is a crystal with a very positive vibration; it encourages optimism and gives energy for new growth in life. It is a very useful crystal to carry with you during times of life change, such as moving home, starting education or a new job, or beginning a new relationship. Aventurine's beautiful green energy with its sparkles of light encourages positive emotional, mental, and spiritual growth.

Fresh starts

In crystal healing, aventurine is placed over the Heart Chakra to ease any fear or anxiety about embracing change or new directions in life. Its gentle energy soothes and calms nervous tension and encourages confidence in new decisions. It can also be placed over the Heart Chakra or Throat Chakra to strengthen and support the entire body after an

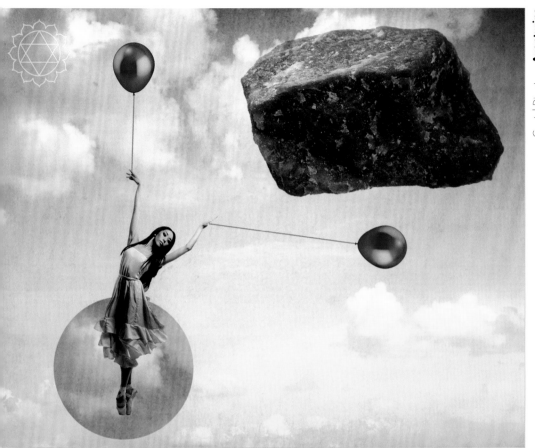

episode of cold or flu, to stimulate energetic restoration and regeneration.

If you are feeling generally tired and depleted, holding aventurine or putting a piece under your pillow at night are simple ways to experience its gentle rejuvenating effect. Placing a piece of aventurine in a warm bath is also very comforting, allowing you to absorb its soothing support though the water.

Diopside

Crystal facts

Hardness
5–6

Color
Mostly golden green;
black pieces can also be found

Geographical sources
Austria, Finland, Germany, Italy,
Russia, US, South Africa

Rarity
Fairly rare; source from
specialist suppliers

Form and structure
Forms as short prismatic-shaped
crystals, clusters, chunks, or blades

Chemical name
Calcium magnesium silicate

Diopside is an unusual crystal that sometimes occurs in twinned form, meaning double crystals forming together. It is most often pale or golden green in color and has a semitransparent appearance resembling glass. It is also dichroic, meaning that it will reflect two colors, for example, green and yellow.

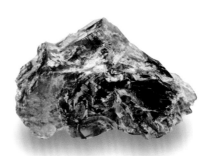

The pale green color of most diopside pieces connects it to the green healing ray of the Heart Chakra. Diopside also shows strong striations, that is, parallel lines running through the crystal structure. This enables diopside to function as a strong channel, moving energy through the Heart Chakra, dissolving any stuck feelings or emotions. Placed over the heart, diopside benefits people who are unable to make decisions in their relationships. It clears the energy and enables a better emotional perspective.

Living energy

Green diopside stimulates a connection to nature and planet Earth, to the green energy that sustains all life. Meditate with a piece of diopside to feel that connection within your Heart Chakra, then go outside

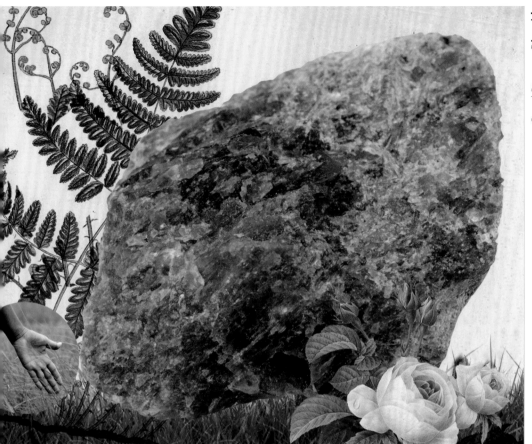

and touch the ground, touch leaves and flowers, and sense the expansion of energy in your hands.

When diopside has a golden-green color, this crystal will help balance the Solar Plexus Chakra just under the ribcage with the Heart Chakra above it. The Solar Plexus Chakra is the place of personal will, which can sometimes become selfish; it needs to be balanced by the loving energy of the Heart Chakra to stay aware of the needs of others. Placing or holding golden-green diopside over the upper abdomen helps to balance these two chakras.

Hiddenite

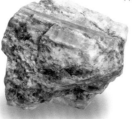

Crystal facts

Hardness
6–7

Color
Pale apple-green

Geographical sources
**Brazil, Myanmar, US,
Madagascar**

Rarity
**Fairly rare; obtain from
specialist suppliers**

Form and structure
**Forms in bladed layers with
vertical cleavage (meaning
it breaks vertically)**

Chemical name
Lithium aluminum silicate

Hiddenite is a member of a mineral family called spodumene, which also includes kunzite (see pages 132–3). These are interesting bladed crystals with a tendency to shatter along vertical lines, so be careful not to drop a piece onto a hard surface. Hiddenite is named after the man who first found it: W.E. Hidden of North Carolina, United States, who discovered it in the nineteenth century.

Hiddenite has a unique pale green color and a soft sheen. This crystal is linked to the Heart Chakra because of its green color. Its energy is very subtle; it acts gently, supporting the emotions when they are in a delicate state. When it is too difficult to express inner feelings, hiddenite simply nurtures the Heart Chakra until it is ready to open. It is placed over the heart in a healing layout to provide a nourishing charge, just working quietly. Hiddenite is also used in healing to awaken gratitude for all the good things we receive in our lives.

Appreciating the good

Meditate with or focus on a piece of hiddenite and practice counting your blessings: opening your heart to gratitude is a wonderfully beneficial exercise with

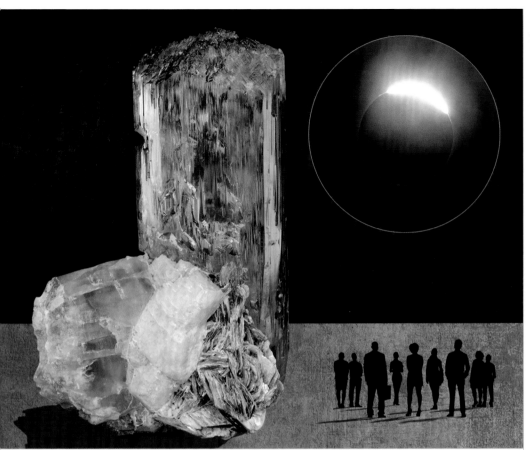

positive potential in your life. Speak your thanks aloud; this makes the energy more powerful. The presence of hiddenite's gentle green ray will support you. As you do this exercise regularly, the feeling of gratitude opens up all kinds of possibilities in your life. Hiddenite helps you to realize your own worth, to receive all the energy that wants to manifest through you, and to feel the best way to go forward.

Kunzite

Crystal facts

Hardness
6–7

Color
Pale pink

Geographical sources
Brazil, Canada, US

Rarity
Fairly rare; obtain from specialist suppliers

Form and structure
Forms as prismatic crystals with vertical striations

Chemical name
Lithium aluminum silicate

Kunzite belongs to a group of minerals called spodumenes, which also includes hiddenite, (see pages 130–1). Spodumenes form in very defined layers with vertical striations (lines), and shatter easily along those vertical lines to form thin sheets or flakes. Because of this fragility it is very difficult to cut or shape; as a result, it is rare to find it in jewelry. Kunzite will fade in the sun, so keep it in the shade to preserve the lovely pink color. It displays a beautiful play of light when turned to different angles, and kunzite has a sparkle which looks quite different to rose quartz (see pages 116–7).

Kunzite links to the pale pink healing ray of divine love and compassion for all beings. This healing ray of divine love is always there, never changing; we are the ones who cut ourselves off from its gentle nurturing support, through our lack of belief and our negative emotions. Kunzite helps to open the inner door and bring back a sense of its presence. Placed over the Heart Chakra in a healing layout, kunzite brings a feeling of gentle light and inner peace.

Finding better days

Kunzite also helps to ease stress, anxiety, or nervous tension, helping to open the heart to feel again, especially after times

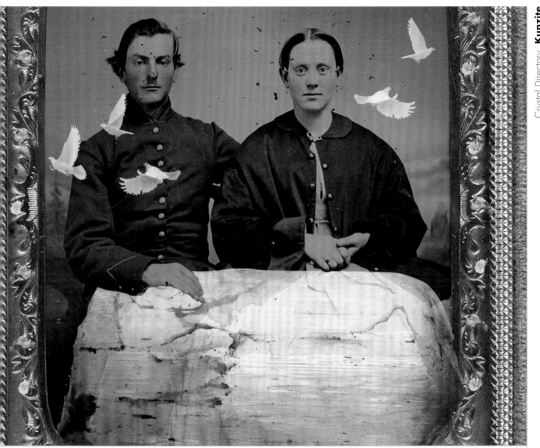

of emotional turmoil. This helps to create a sense of renewal and purpose, a feeling that it is safe to trust in and follow your heart. It is good to meditate with or focus on kunzite on a regular basis as you begin to move forward again in your life.

Moss Agate

Crystal facts

Hardness
6.5

Color
**Pale green background
with dark green inclusions**

Geographical sources
India, Middle East, US

Rarity
Widely available

Form and structure
**Forms in masses and
layered deposits**

Chemical name
Silicon dioxide

In mineralogical terms, moss agate is incorrectly named: it does not have bands running through it like true agate, but is actually a kind of chalcedony. The name, however, is a common one that has stuck to this particular stone. Moss agate is a type of microcrystalline quartz with a pale, semitranslucent background and many tiny inclusions of dark green minerals that give it its name. If you hold a piece to the light, the green inclusions really do have a plantlike appearance.

Moss agate's appearance links it to the abundance of life on our planet. It encourages a connection to nature, to the energy and vitality of green growing plant life. It is a good stone to carry if you live or work in a predominantly urban environment; moss agate helps you to stay connected to the green ray of vibrant nature. As it encourages inner calm and balance, many people find it a very positive stone to work with. Its wide availability in raw or cut and polished forms, such as palm stones, spheres, or tumblestones, makes it a popular choice of crystal for a starter's collection.

Touching base

In crystal healing, moss agate can be placed over the Heart Chakra in the center of the chest to release old

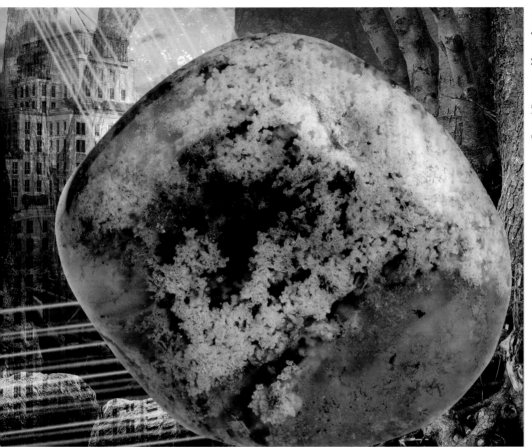

emotional blockages and encourage new and better connections to the environment and to other people. Placed over the Root Chakra at the base of the spine, moss agate encourages a deep connection to Earth, bringing a sense of inner grounding and stability. It is also used to help regenerate the auric field around the body when energy is very depleted or the person is physically exhausted; holding a piece of moss agate in each hand helps to restore inner vitality.

Citrine

Crystal facts

Hardness
7

Color
Pale translucent yellow

Geographical sources
**US, Canada, Mexico,
Russia, Europe**

Rarity
Widely available

Form and structure
**Forms in points, clusters,
or layered deposits**

Chemical name
Silicon dioxide

Citrine is golden quartz, colored thanks to traces of iron being present when the crystal formed. When buying citrine take care that the stone is genuine; very bright yellow and white stones sold as citrine are likely to be heat-treated amethyst. If you are looking for citrine for crystal healing purposes it is especially important to buy genuine pieces of high quality.

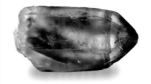

Citrine is the form of quartz used to stimulate energy in the Solar Plexus Chakra, found just under the middle of the rib cage. This energy center symbolizes personal power and manifestation of success; if citrine is placed or held directly over the Solar Plexus Chakra, it will regenerate and amplify the energy in this area. It is important to focus clearly on the kind of success you want, or the aspects of your life where you would like energy to increase: as with all energy work, your intention guides the result. It is particularly useful to meditate with citrine or carry it with you if you are changing jobs or life direction, as it helps to clarify your new path.

Helping yourself thrive

In Feng Shui, all golden objects are considered to attract wealth. Try placing

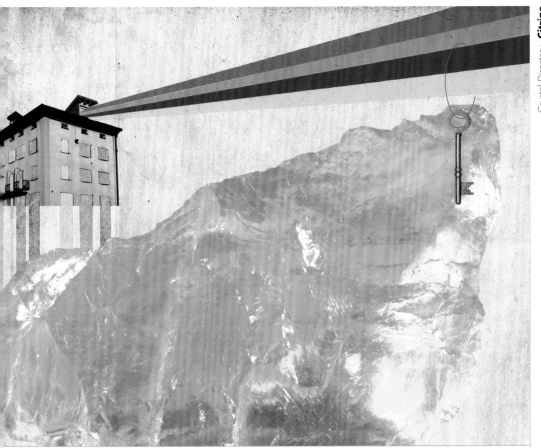

a medium-sized piece of citrine in the northwest corner of your home, the area of abundance and prosperity, to allow citrine's energy of manifestation to work in your space.

In crystal healing, citrine is also used to clear energy that may have stagnated or become blocked in the person's auric field. This can be negative thought patterns or ideas that persistently prevent someone from making progress in life. Placing citrine over the Solar Plexus Chakra or the Sacral Chakra just below the navel dissolves negativity and restores positive beliefs.

Chrysoprase

Crystal facts

Hardness
7

Color
**Pale turquoise green with
black swirls or specks**

Geographical sources
**Brazil, Australia, Madagascar,
South Africa, Russia**

Rarity
Widely available

Form and structure
**Forms as chunky granular deposits
or nodules in rock layers**

Chemical name
Silicon dioxide

Chrysoprase is one of the rarer forms of microcrystalline quartz; its unique pale turquoise-green color comes from nickel. Raw pieces have a granular appearance, but when the stone is polished the color becomes beautifully semitransparent. Chrysoprase needs to be kept away from strong sunlight, which bleaches and fades the color. It is easily available as polished tumblestones; larger pieces can be carved into statues or spheres where the color really stands out.

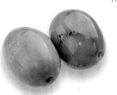

In crystal healing, chrysoprase is associated with attracting abundance. This can mean money, but it can also mean positive energy of any kind. Abundance cannot be grabbed, it has to flow into your life; from a healing perspective, keeping the Heart Chakra open is key to this. Placing chrysoprase over the Heart Chakra or holding a piece in each hand helps to loosen and liberate any blocked energy which is preventing a person from receiving abundance.

Open to opportunity

Meditating or holding chrysoprase brings a sense of expansion and vitality, like holding your arms wide and taking a deep breath. It is a good crystal to carry with you if you want to maintain a wider perspective. It helps to loosen restricted

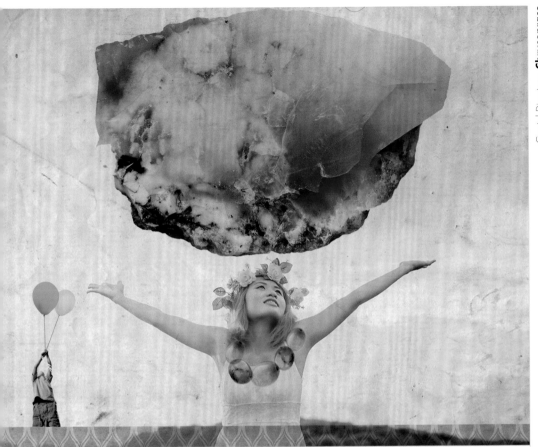

thinking and keeps you open to new possibilities where you can literally "put your heart" into something. To find such opportunities, your heart has to be open to receive them. Chrysoprase is a wonderful crystal companion in times of change.

Finding romance

Chrysoprase is also a lovely crystal to wear or to carry to attract the energy of love. If you have not had a relationship for some time and you would like this to change, then chrysoprase can help, again by opening your Heart Chakra to receive new possibilities and new people into your life.

Emerald

Crystal facts

Hardness
7.5–8

Color
Deep vivid green

Geographical sources
**Africa, Columbia,
Brazil, Russia**

Rarity
**Top-quality pieces are rare gems;
lower-grade stones are readily
available for healing**

Form and structure
Forms as hexagonal crystals

Chemical name
Beryllium aluminum silicate

Emeralds are one of the most beautiful and rare of all precious stones. The best-quality pieces have a uniquely vivid, rich green color, thanks to the presence of chromium and iron. These gems are members of the beryl family of stones; their hardness makes them suitable for cutting and faceting. True emerald stones contain what look like tiny imperfections called inclusions; if they look too clear and perfect, they are probably fake.

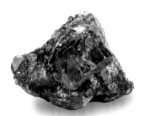

Emeralds have to be kept carefully; they are treated with oil to protect them, and if the stones are washed too much they may dry out and shatter. Gem-quality emeralds are reserved for jewelry making; however, pieces of lower-grade mineral that form around them, called green beryl, are available through crystal suppliers. Sometimes pieces of green beryl may have tiny crystallized emeralds in them.

A benevolent Earth

In crystal healing, emerald is another green crystal that links to the Heart Chakra. It is striking how many green stones there are; this shows how often the mineral energy of the Earth links to us, manifesting its loving communication through the green healing ray. Emerald crystal energy links us to the heart of nature, the heart of the Earth; it bathes

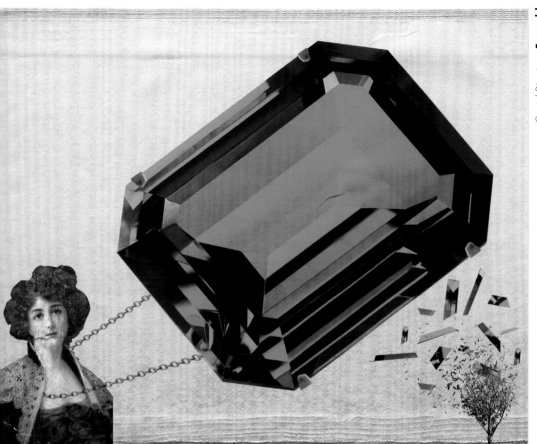

and nourishes the Heart Chakra. It triggers the feeling of compassion, unconditional love, for all of nature and all beings.

Accepting good fortune

Emerald also attracts abundance. Wear it or carry it with you to open your heart to receive all the positive energy that wants to flow into your life. Learning to receive, being truly open and receptive, is quite an art: it means trusting that whatever you truly seek is on its way to you. Meditate with emerald and focus on its vivid green color to be ready to receive.

Garnet

Crystal facts

Hardness
7

Color
**Rich ruby red to dark
red or brown**

Geographical sources
**India, Sri Lanka, US,
Africa, Brazil**

Rarity
Widely available

Form and structure
**Forms as twelve-sided crystals with
lozenge-shaped facets**

Chemical name
**Aluminum silicate or
calcium silicate**

There are many types and colors of garnet; the stone forms in volcanic rocks all over the world. The two most commonly known types are pyrope garnets, the small, teardrop-shaped gleaming garnets most often used in jewelry, and almandine garnets, which are larger and heavier with a dark red color; the latter type is used in crystal healing. The name "garnet" is linked to the pomegranate, because the gleaming red seeds of this fruit look like small, gleaming, red jewels.

Although garnets are considered inferior to rubies because they are cheaper, this is not a fair assessment: garnets have a beautiful red energy all of their own. The pomegranate is a fruit associated with fertility, abundance, and life energy. These are also the qualities of garnet, which supports the feminine qualities of birth, creativity, and nurturing. Both pyrope and almandine garnets are good to carry or wear as jewelry in order to encourage fertility. Garnet works with the Root Chakra at the base of the spine, which links to the womb—the source of life and creative energy. Garnet warms and revitalizes the reproductive system, and is a good stone to carry or meditate with during menstruation, to feel supported and connected to the Earth during this time.

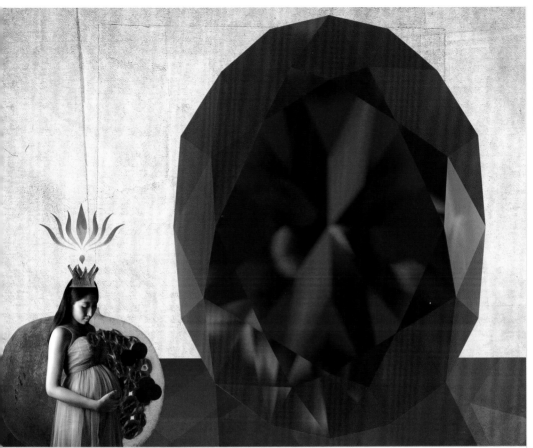

Grounding yourself

In crystal healing, garnet can be placed over the pubic bone at the level of the Root Chakra, between the knees, or over the base of the spine if the person receiving treatment lies on their front. In any of these positions garnet will work to energize and replenish the Root Chakra. Garnet can be used to enhance this energy in men as well as women; in men it brings a feeling of being nourished, grounded, and centered.

Amethyst

Crystal facts

Hardness
7

Color
Ranges from pale to deepest purple

Geographical sources
US, Mexico, Brazil, Africa, Canada

Rarity
Widely available

Form and structure
Forms as six-sided crystals with faceted points; also as clusters of smaller crystals or masses of tiny crystals enclosed in a bubble of volcanic rock called a geode

Chemical name
Silicon dioxide

Amethyst is one of the most striking crystals in the quartz group, radiating beautiful shades of purple. The color arises because varying amounts of iron or aluminum combine with silicon dioxide during the formation of the crystals. Amethyst can occur in a whole host of different shapes, sizes, and shades. Larger, darker-colored pieces or geodes can be expensive, but amethyst is also available as small, inexpensive, polished tumblestones. There is an amethyst for everyone.

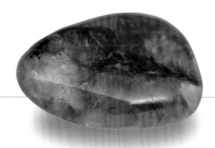

Choosing amethyst is very much a case of letting your eyes travel over all the different hues of the stones, feeling which one is right for you. Your eye might be drawn to the deepest violet purple, or to a much softer, lighter shade. Purple is a deeply soothing and healing color, and the sheer variety of shades in amethyst is amazing. Seeing all the different shapes that amethyst can take is also important.

Again, you will be drawn to the structure that feels right to you.

Amethyst & the spirit

In crystal healing, amethyst is used to restore the Crown Chakra at the top of the head: when energized, this chakra expands spiritual awareness. Amethyst

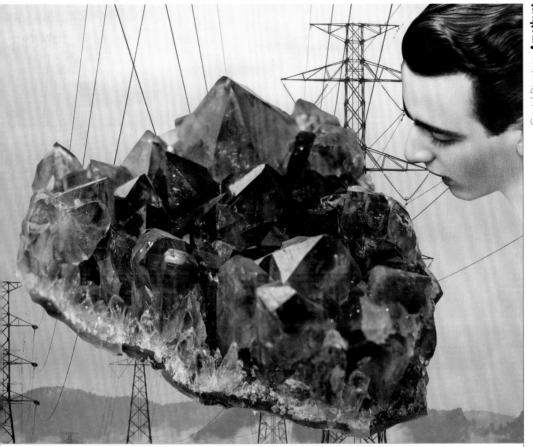

also offers protection to the entire human energy field from any negative influences in the environment. It soothes and calms the brain and relieves mental stress or overload, and is very beneficial to the nervous system, helping to calm anxiety and restore inner peace.

Amethyst also opens a connection to personal spiritual guides or guardian angels through its gentle purple ray.

Meditating with amethyst, either by focusing on or holding a crystal, is a useful practice to facilitate awareness of inner vision and soul purpose.

Spirit Quartz

Crystal facts

Hardness
7

Color
Very pale lilac

Geographical sources
South Africa

Rarity
**Rarer than amethyst,
so more expensive**

Form and structure
**Forms in candle shapes
with very defined terminations,
and sides coated with many
tiny crystals**

Chemical name
Silicon dioxide

Spirit quartz is a fascinating variety of quartz very similar to amethyst, discovered only recently in South Africa. It has gained popularity in crystal healing because of its very finely-tuned energy. As you look at a piece of spirit quartz, it sparkles all over with light because the sides of the formation are covered in thousands of miniature individual crystals. Most spirit quartz has a unique pale lilac amethyst hue, though some clear or yellow (citrine) quartz types have been found.

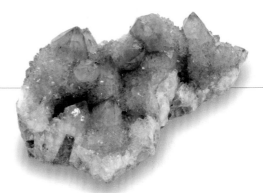

Holding or observing spirit quartz shows you light in motion, a sparkling energy that is refreshing, spontaneous, and free. The multidirectional structure of this rare quartz lifts the heart and eases the mind, pointing to a world of infinite possibilities. The many tiny crystals clustered around the structure of a piece are like a community, showing that the presence of many can unite as one, to radiate light and energy.

The spirit of togetherness

In crystal healing, spirit quartz is used to stimulate a cooperative attitude in people who tend to be isolated. It acts as a reminder that we all need other people,

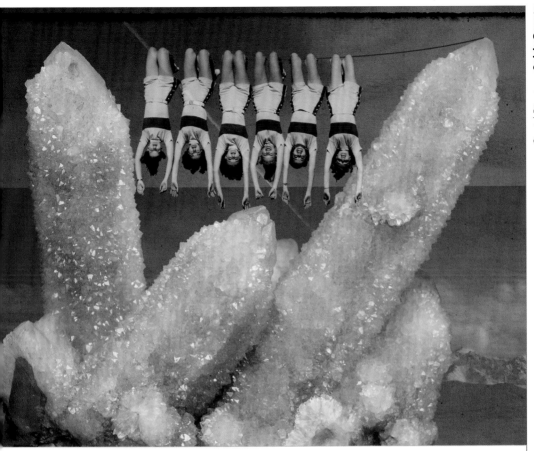

that we are more effective as a group than when we act alone. The sparkling radiance of spirit quartz encourages us to connect with others, to share our energy and unite in a common purpose. It also connects us with our own spiritual community of guides and angels, to know our soul's purpose.

Place spirit quartz in your home, particularly in the living room where the "hearth" or "heart" of your space is; it will encourage and support positive and harmonious relationships with your family and friends.

Sugilite

Crystal facts

Hardness
6–6.5

Color
**Deep violet with pale
lilac and black specks**

Geographical sources
Japan, Canada, South Africa

Rarity
**Rare; obtain from
specialist crystal suppliers**

Form and structure
Forms in layered deposits

Chemical name
**Potassium sodium lithium iron
manganese aluminum silicate**

Sugilite is named for the Japanese geologist Ken-ichi Sugi, who first discovered it in the mid-twentieth century. Its distinctive rich purple color is opaque and dense, with tiny black or paler lilac specks or dots. The deeper the purple color, the more expensive it is to buy. Sugilite is sought after by mineral collectors, so it is fairly rare and needs to be obtained from specialist suppliers. Raw pieces are sometimes available, and when sugilite is polished its violet shade is even more beautiful. It can be found carved and polished into spheres,

eggs, or palm stones to hold; it is also set in silver jewelry.

The deep violet shade of sugilite connects it to the Crown Chakra at the top of the head. The Crown Chakra resonates to two color energy frequencies: luminous, shining white, which links to the stars; and

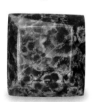

deep, radiant violet, which links to the angelic realms. The deep violet of sugilite makes it a stone for spiritual awakening. It encourages the violet energy ray to radiate through the Crown Chakra; this is a deeply healing and soothing energy, gently dissolving all blocked or stagnant places in the auric field, bathing body, mind, and spirit in peace.

A spiritual shield

Wearing or carrying sugilite is also a form of protection; its violet energy surrounds

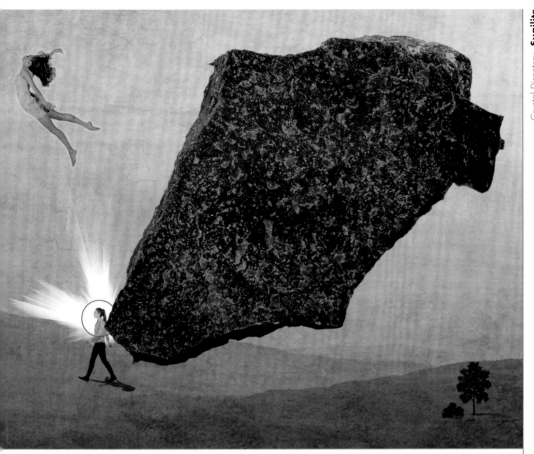

the body like an invisible cloak wherever you go. It is a reminder that you are more than your body; you have a spiritual identity as well. Meditate or focus on sugilite whenever you need to find a higher perspective in your life.

In crystal layouts, sugilite can be placed over the Crown Chakra or the Third Eye Chakra in the middle of the forehead to open higher energy frequencies. It soothes people who are nervous or highly strung, and helps those who have problems sleeping.

Seraphinite

Crystal facts

Hardness
2–2.5

Color
Dark green and silvery-white

Geographical sources
Russia

Rarity
Fairly rare; obtain from specialist suppliers

Form and structure
Forms as granular layers

Chemical name
Magnesium iron aluminum silicate hydroxide

Seraphinite is an unusual dark green crystal with interlaced shimmering silvery-white streaks; these take on feathery shapes, so they look like angels' wings. The name seraphinite comes from the word "seraph," which means angel. Seraphinite is a relative newcomer to

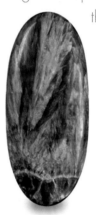

the crystal healing world; it was discovered in Siberia in Russia toward the end of the twentieth century. Seraphinite is very soft; with a hardness of only around 2, it can easily be scratched, even with a fingernail, so keep it carefully.

Seraphinite, as its name and appearance suggest, is used to facilitate communication with the angelic kingdom. The idea of having a guardian angel is familiar to many; using seraphinite in meditation, either focusing on or holding a piece of the crystal, is a gentle and simple way to feel more connected to your particular angel's energy. If you place a piece of seraphinite under your pillow, your dreams may bring you insights into the angelic realms.

Embracing divine love

The colors in seraphinite link it to the Heart Chakra (green) and the Crown Chakra (white). Seraphinite helps to connect these two chakras, bringing spiritual awareness from the Crown into the level of the Heart. This allows higher spiritual levels of love to

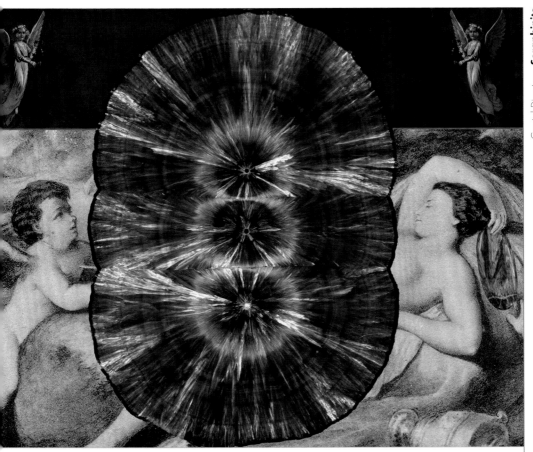

be received into the Heart Chakra, and as this energy builds, it automatically radiates out into the world. In crystal layouts, seraphinite may be placed on either or both of these chakras to enhance this effect. It has become popular as a crystal set in silver jewelry but can also be sourced from crystal suppliers in raw or polished form. Wearing or carrying seraphinite helps you to be a messenger of light, quietly carrying the radiance of love wherever you go.

Pietersite

Crystal facts

Hardness
7

Color
**Dark blue, brown, and
gold bands**

Geographical sources
South Africa, China

Rarity
**Fairly rare; obtain from
specialist crystal suppliers**

Form and structure
Forms in layered deposits

Chemical name
Silicon dioxide

Pietersite is an example of a crystal that has only recently been discovered and come into use in crystal healing. It was originally found in South Africa, but deposits have also been found in China. This is a very unusual form of microcrystalline quartz, in which layers of different mineral-rich sands have been fused and squeezed together over millions of years, creating different colored layers that reflect light back at each other. Pietersite has quite a dark appearance until you turn it to the light, when you see blue, gold, and gray reflections.

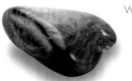

The main colors in pietersite relate to the Third Eye Chakra (dark blue) and the Solar Plexus Chakra (gold). Pietersite links these two chakras to unite personal will from the latter with the cosmic view of the former. Often, if you insist on seeing things only from a limited perspective, you limit what could happen; pietersite balances what you want with a wider field of possibility—the elusive and expansive power of the universe. Expect the unexpected when you meditate or focus with pietersite.

Finding new paths

If you are undertaking guided meditation journeys to explore your own field of possibility, then hold pietersite or place it either on the Third Eye Chakra or the Solar Plexus Chakra. It can be interesting

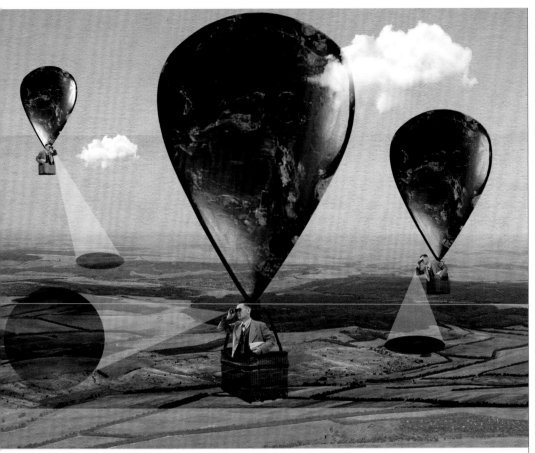

to see which chakra feels more responsive
to pietersite; let your intuition guide you.
Pietersite is a great stone to work with
as a spiritual activator to stimulate new
directions and visions in your life.

Selenite

Crystal facts

Hardness
2

Color
Milky white

Geographical sources
Obtained from Mexico

Rarity
Widely available

Form and structure
Forms as flat-faced, tabular, block, or bladed crystals

Chemical name
Hydrated calcium sulfate

Selenite is a translucent crystal with an ethereal and gentle presence. It has a strongly vertical structure and visible vertical lines; as a result it splits easily into long, straight pieces. This is a very soft crystal with a tendency to shatter or break, so handle it with care. Selenite forms in caves around hot springs, solidifying out of mineralized water containing calcium sulfate; sometimes, pieces can be obtained with bubbles of water still visible inside. Large pieces are often called "wands" or "swords" because of their elongated shape.

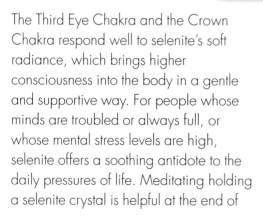

The Third Eye Chakra and the Crown Chakra respond well to selenite's soft radiance, which brings higher consciousness into the body in a gentle and supportive way. For people whose minds are troubled or always full, or whose mental stress levels are high, selenite offers a soothing antidote to the daily pressures of life. Meditating holding a selenite crystal is helpful at the end of a crazy day to bring a cool, calm sense of peace to the mind.

Brightening up your aura

The wand-like shape of selenite makes it a very popular crystal healing tool. In the hands of a crystal healer, a wand can be used to "channel" energy, meaning to enable energy to pass freely into or out of the body. Selenite wands are used to

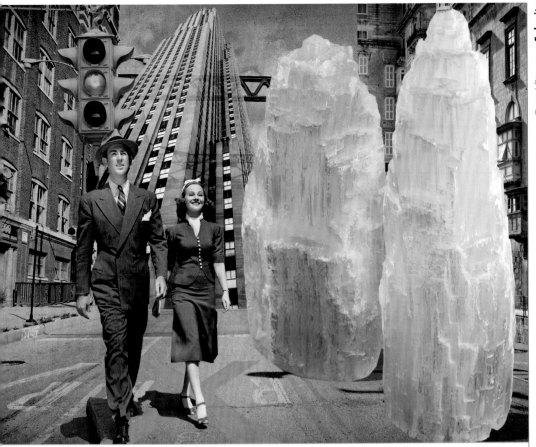

"spring clean" the auric field; they draw
negativity up and out of the system with a
sparkling and refreshing sensation. Many
crystal healers work with selenite wands
fused with other crystals to enhance their
channeling power. In crystal healing
layouts, long blades of selenite may be
laid on the body to channel negativity out
of a particular area, or to restore energy
flow to blocked chakras.

Ametrine

Crystal facts

Hardness
7

Color
**Purple and pale
yellow combination**

Geographical sources
Uruguay and Bolivia

Rarity
**Somewhat scarce;
consult specialist suppliers**

Form and structure
**Forms as six-sided terminated
crystals or clusters**

Chemical name
Silicon dioxide

Ametrine is an unusual form of quartz in which amethyst and citrine form together and combine in swirling bands of purple and pale yellow. This creates a flowing and subtle play of color, especially when you hold the crystal to the light. Ametrine is sold in raw form but often shaped and polished to bring out the colors. It is also used in high-quality jewelry.

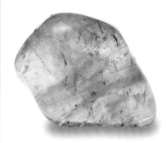

The natural fusion of amethyst and citrine combines the properties of both crystals in one, making ametrine a unique stone to use in healing. The spiritually expansive qualities of amethyst combine with the energizing qualities of citrine. This makes ametrine a wonderful crystal to work with during times of personal transformation, especially those linked to spiritual awakening. At such moments, energy is needed to support the process of change you are undergoing; citrine offers this support while amethyst continues the expansion. Ametrine is a catalyst for personal change.

Seeing the bigger picture

Ametrine works to balance the energies of spirituality and personal power so that both work together for the highest good.

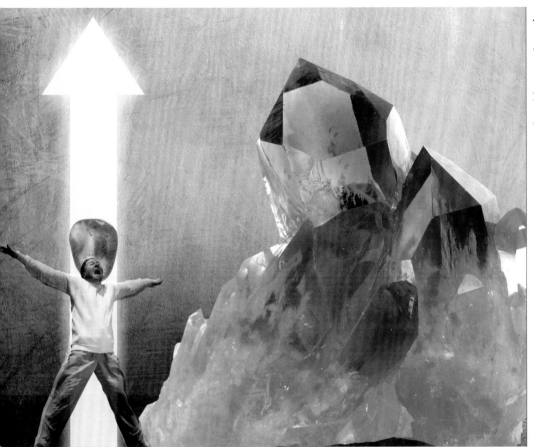

Instead of energy expansion being only for personal gain, ametrine enables higher awareness to influence choices so that the very best potential can be achieved. Hence, wearing or carrying ametrine in daily life acts as a reminder that success can have a spiritual aspect as well as a physical manifestation.

In crystal healing, Ametrine works well placed over the top of the head (the Crown Chakra) or over the Solar Plexus Chakra just under the rib cage. In either position it will balance the purple (spiritual) and gold (solar energy) rays so the whole energy field is resonant with potential. It is a beautiful crystal to meditate with to feel more in touch with a higher spiritual purpose in life.

Apophyllite

Crystal facts

Hardness
4–5

Color
**Most common as clear crystals;
also green**

Geographical sources
**India, Greenland, Iceland,
Canada**

Rarity
**Clear type is widely
available; green is rarer**

Form and structure
**Forms as cubic or
pyramid-shaped crystals**

Chemical name
**Hydrated potassium
calcium silicate**

Apophyllite crystals are most often clear, and sometimes sold with pale pink stilbite crystals attached since both crystals often form together. Clusters are common, with very clear sparkling end terminations and defined lozenge-shaped facets. Compared to clear quartz, apophyllite shimmers with a brighter luster. Smaller crystals often sit on wide columnar-shaped pieces. It is a medium-priced crystal to buy as a quality piece, but small-end terminations are often sold separately and are very affordable. Green apophyllite is rarer and is sought after by mineral collectors.

Clear apophyllite opens channels to the spiritual awareness of angels, fairies, and devic beings (small spirits who guard plant life). It brings a sense of radiating lightness. One of the best ways to experience apophyllite is to observe a crystal in meditation; as you concentrate on its form, allow your awareness to travel inside its structure, as into a crystal cave of possibility or a temple of light.

Playful energy

Apophyllite supports the inner child, the part of all of us that retains the memory of curiosity, lightness, spontaneity, and living in the moment with a fascination for all that is new. Many of us have forgotten what it is like to be in that space of eternal discovery; adult life tends to swamp this kind of spontaneous and creative energy. If you want to re-open your own creative

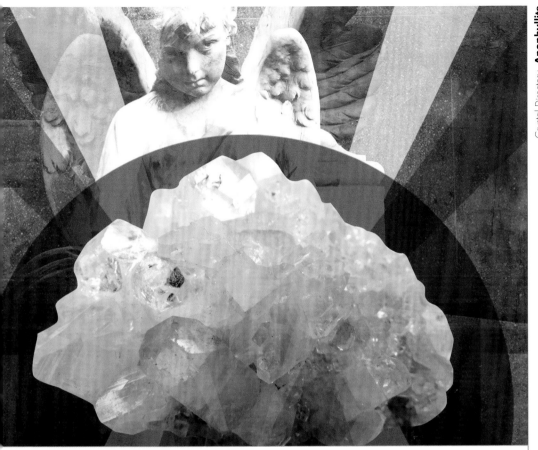

potential and your ability to express it, then meditate with apophyllite, or carry a small piece with you during your day.

Pieces of clear apophyllite work well placed above the head in a healing layout to encourage the opening of the Crown Chakra, and to increase awareness of a person's spiritual guide or guardian angel.

Celestite

Crystal facts

Hardness
3–3.5

Color
Mostly pale blue; white, gray
or green types are unusual

Geographical sources
Madagascar, US,
parts of Europe

Rarity
Source from specialist suppliers

Form and structure
Forms in clusters with prismatic
terminations; also geodes (rock
bubbles with small crystals
growing inside)

Chemical name
Strontium sulfate

Celestite (sometimes called celestine by suppliers) is a lovely but fragile crystal with a tendency to shatter; clusters with terminations need to be kept carefully or the tips will break off. The color most widely available is a pale blue-gray shade, which has an icy translucence; quality pieces have a slightly shimmering appearance. Celestite is not always easy to find, and may require visits to specialist suppliers or crystal fairs. Clusters or geodes are the most commonly available pieces.

The energy of celestite is very pure, light, and elevated. It makes you think of mountains, of high spaces where the energy is open, clear, cool, and expansive. Celestite works with the higher energies of the Throat, Third Eye, and Crown Chakras, opening communication with wider levels of spiritual awareness, as well as angelic and personal guides.

It enhances meditation by encouraging stillness and clarity of intention; however, the quality of its energy is also soft, like clouds or mist, offering a gentle way of being transported to the higher realms. Meditating with celestite, either holding or focusing on a piece of the crystal, soothes and calms the eyes as you look at its gentle blue-gray color.

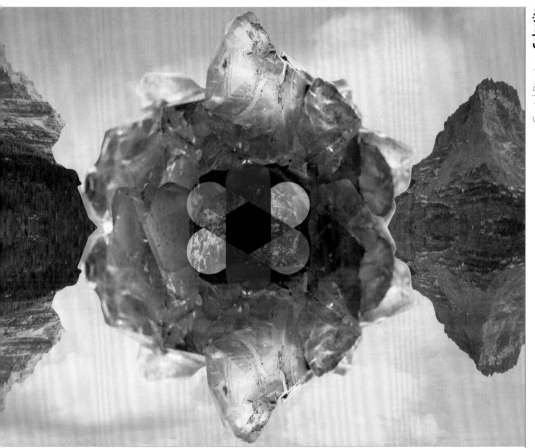

Guiding dreams

Placing celestite in your bedroom is a good way to promote peaceful sleep, as well as open dream-time communication with your angelic and spiritual guides. It also offers protection against environmental or electromagnetic stress while you sleep. If you want an answer to a question that is important in your life, ask it out loud before you fall asleep within celestite's radiance, then see what happens when you wake up: you may be surprised by the message!

Charoite

Crystal facts

Hardness
6

Color
Pale purple mixed with white, gray, black, and gold specks

Geographical sources
Russia

Rarity
Fairly unusual; obtain from specialist suppliers

Form and structure
Forms in complex mixed fibrous crystal layers

Chemical name
Hydrated potassium sodium calcium barium strontium silicate hydroxide fluoride

As you can tell from the extremely long chemical name, charoite is a crystal that is made up of a complicated cocktail of chemical elements. It formed when layers of limestone were infused with alkaline-rich minerals in the presence of extreme heat. When you look at a piece of charoite, you see purple mixed with white, gray, and black layers; it is like looking into a swirling mix of colored paints. Charoite is only found in Russia and takes its name from the Chara river in Siberia.

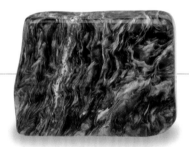

The purple color of charoite links it to the Crown Chakra, the energy center at the top of the head that opens the gateway to spiritual awakening and awareness of higher energy frequencies. Because charoite also contains other colors (white, gray, black, and gold), it is seen as a transmuting crystal, able to gather up fears, anxieties, and negative thoughts and transform them into creative and inspirational energy patterns. In crystal healing it is often placed over the Third Eye Chakra in the center of the forehead or above the head to stimulate the Crown Chakra. It can also be placed over the Heart Chakra to align the heart with spiritual truth.

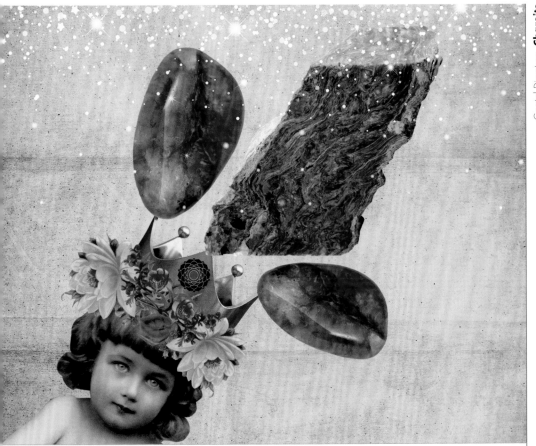

Mind & spirit

Charoite also helps to anchor spiritual
energy into the body, particularly when
the mind has doubts and gets in the way.
Holding or meditating with a piece of
charoite helps you accept the flow of divine
energy into the physical frame of your
body, where it interacts with all the chakra
centers. It brings a sparkling sense of
inner light and peace.

Danburite

Crystal facts

Hardness
7–7.5

Color
**Mostly transparent or
white; very rare examples are
pale yellow or pink**

Geographical sources
**US, Switzerland, Myanmar,
Mexico**

Rarity
**Fairly rare; obtain from
specialist suppliers**

Form and structure
**Forms as prismatic crystals
with a diamond-shaped cross-
section and vertical striations**

Chemical name
Calcium borosilicate

Danburite crystals are usually four-sided, clear or semitransparent with wedge-shaped terminations. In clear pieces, light refracts to form soft rainbow reflections. It can be found in bladed shapes up to 12 inches (30 cm) long. Its four-sided structure shows it is different from quartz, which has a six-sided structure. Danburite is also lighter in weight than quartz. When polished, danburite has a smooth, silky feel to its surface.

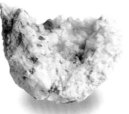

Danburite is one of a group of new crystals to appear on the crystal healing list, after it gained popularity toward the end of the twentieth century. Danburite was originally sourced from Danbury in Connecticut, United States, after which it is named, but it has since been found in other locations such as Switzerland.

In crystal healing, the availability of new and different crystals is a sign that the Earth is yielding these healing gifts to help humanity in its current path.

Peaceful insight

The clear and light presence of danburite links to very high-energy frequencies and spiritual awareness. It opens and expands the Crown Chakra at the top of the head to receive deep spiritual guidance. Placed on the forehead over the Third

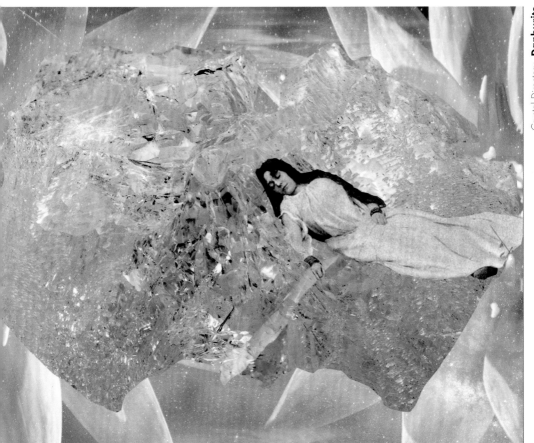

Eye Chakra or over the top of the head, danburite gently assists this opening to higher and angelic energies. The key word is gentle; some crystals can be powerful in their brilliance, but danburite acts in a supportive way to assist opening at a pace that is right for you.

Holding or meditating with a Danburite crystal opens your psychic perception and may give you impressions or information that you were not expecting; however, remember this is happening to support your spiritual expansion.

Diamond

Crystal facts

Hardness
10

Color
**In its rough state, cream or beige
and opaque; brilliantly clear when
cut and polished; very rare black,
blue, or yellow examples exist**

Geographical sources
**South Africa, Australia,
Brasil, Russia**

Rarity
**Rare as mineral specimens;
Herkimer diamond (see below)
is used in crystal healing**

Form and structure
**Forms as cuboid or
octahedral crystals**

Chemical name
Carbon

Diamonds are pure carbon, the hardest substance found in nature. They form due to incredibly high temperatures and pressure deep within the Earth's crust. It took more than a billion years for diamonds to take shape; they are among the most ancient of all Earth minerals. Their rarity and their utter brilliance when polished have made them objects of desire and fascination throughout human history; today they often mark rites of passage such as engagements or coming of age.

Pure raw diamonds are not usually available as pieces for use in healing; because of the rarity of diamonds they are preferred for jewelry making. However, there is a kind of crystal with a beautiful, pure, brilliant light that resembles diamond. Known as Herkimer diamonds, they develop inside cavities of dolostone, and are used in crystal healing.

Herkimer diamond

This is not a diamond in the pure carbon sense; it is actually a rare form of quartz, silicon dioxide, with a hardness of 7. Herkimer diamonds form in small, stubby, double-terminated shapes with defined facets, and are only found in the United States. They are called diamonds because of their particular sparkling

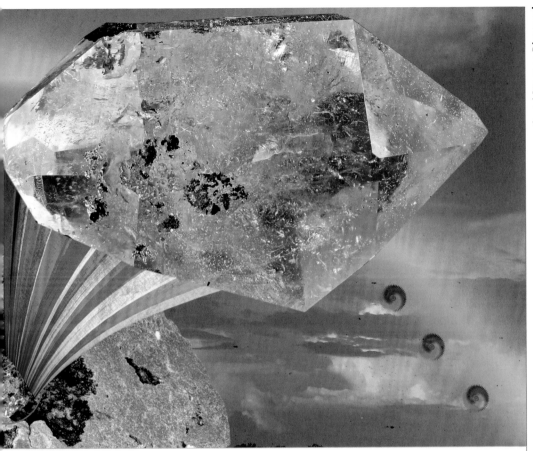

appearance, which is much lighter and brighter than regular clear quartz.

When the energy of diamond is needed in crystal healing, Herkimer diamonds can be used very effectively. They open the Crown Chakra and expand spiritual awareness; they can also be placed over the Third Eye Chakra in the middle of the forehead to enhance psychic awareness.

Placing a Herkimer diamond in each hand of a person receiving a healing treatment thoroughly energizes and renews that person's energy system because Herkimer diamonds reflect all the colors of the rainbow—the colors of all the chakra energy centers.

Iolite

Crystal facts

Hardness
7–7.5

Color
Deep violet-blue

Geographical sources
**Canada, Sri Lanka, Tanzania,
Myanmar, India**

Rarity
**Raw uncut pieces are rare;
obtain from specialist suppliers**

Form and structure
**Forms as hexagonal
crystals or granular masses
within volcanic rocks**

Chemical name
Magnesium aluminum silicate

Iolite is the crystalline form of the mineral cordierite, which is often found alongside granite rock deposits. It has an unusual deep violet-blue color due to the presence of magnesium. Its hardness means it can be cut and polished; gem-quality pieces can even be faceted to show off the color. Iolite is unusual because when it is polished, it displays an effect called pleochroism, meaning it reflects different colors according to the light, such as violet, blue, pink, or gold.

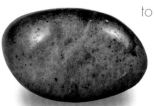

The deep, dark blue color of iolite links it to the Third Eye Chakra in the center of the forehead. The use of iolite in crystal healing depends on the intention of the treatment. On a simple level, placing iolite on the forehead soothes and calms stress, anxiety, or too much mental chatter, bringing a feeling of peace and calm to the mind. On a deeper level, the Third Eye is the psychic chakra, the place where the mind can expand its awareness into visions, dreams, and super-sensory experiences. A meditation focusing on these other realms of awareness can be enhanced by placing a piece of iolite over the Third Eye. The best-quality iolite crystals are used in jewelry but pieces of raw, unpolished iolite are sometimes available through specialist crystal suppliers and can be used in this manner.

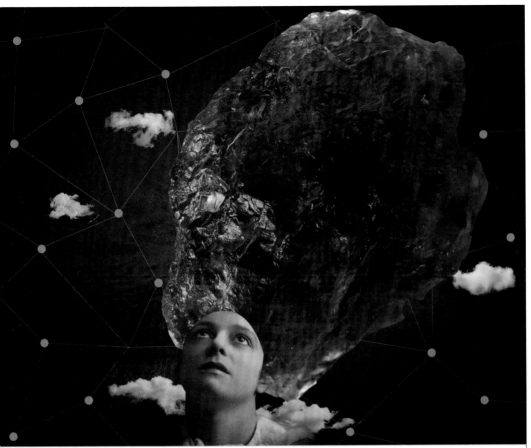

Thinking outside the box

Iolite also stimulates inspiration; it is an excellent crystal to have beside you in the workplace to support creative thinking. Hold a piece of iolite or focus on it to help your thoughts expand in new directions. This crystal encourages a feeling of calm when under pressure; its soothing, cooling energy brings the mind and thoughts back into clarity.

Kyanite

Crystal facts

Hardness
4.5 when scratched parallel to vertical axis; 6.5 when scratched perpendicular to it

Color
Mostly pale blue; rarer forms are white, green, gray, or black

Geographical sources
Africa, India, Switzerland, Russia, US

Rarity
Fairly rare; obtain from specialist suppliers

Form and structure
Forms as long parallel blades with vertical striations

Chemical name
Aluminum silicate

Kyanite is a beautiful pale blue crystal that forms in thin vertical layers like sheets of paper laid on top of each other. It is found alongside granite or other volcanic rock deposits. As with all layered minerals, kyanite tends to shatter along its vertical lines; its hardness varies, so it is weaker along the vertical axis and stronger on the cross axis. Its flat surfaces show a pearl-like sheen when it is turned to different angles under strong light. Kyanite is mainly available as raw unpolished pieces; its peculiar hardness makes it difficult to polish or set in jewelry.

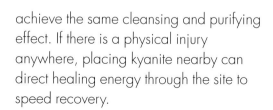

In crystal healing, kyanite works as a conductor, helping to clear places in the auric field where energy is stuck. It also opens the flow and movement of energy through all the chakra centers along the spine. Long blades of kyanite are sometimes used by crystal healers like wands to remove blockages. Placing these blades on the body can also achieve the same cleansing and purifying effect. If there is a physical injury anywhere, placing kyanite nearby can direct healing energy through the site to speed recovery.

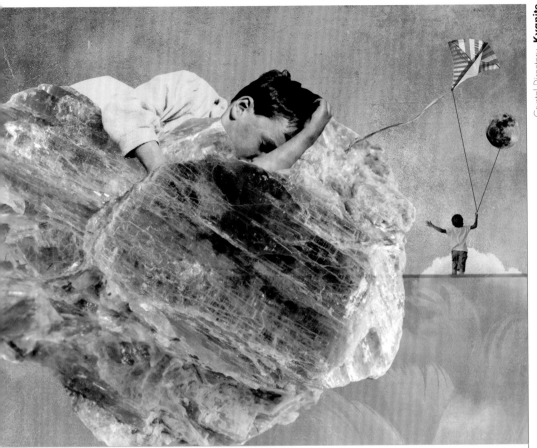

Seeing new visions

Meditating holding kyanite can open up levels of spiritual and psychic awareness; again, kyanite acts like a channel, freeing up perception and opening the mind to new possibilities. If you sleep with a piece of kyanite under your pillow you may experience very unusual and vivid dreams with important messages for you.

Labradorite

Crystal facts

Hardness
6–6.5

Color
Blue-green, with a distinctive blue sheen when turned to the light

Geographical sources
Canada, Finland, Norway, Mexico, Russia

Rarity
Widely available

Form and structure
Forms as blocks or massed deposits within volcanic rocks

Chemical name
Calcium sodium aluminum silicate

Labradorite was named after the Labrador Peninsula in Canada, where the mineral was first found in the eighteenth century. It is a kind of feldspar mineral; these are found all over the world within the Earth's crust. Labradorite is remarkable because as the stone is turned toward strong light, it shows a play of vivid color, usually a shimmering blue; this display happens because light rays are being mirrored back and forth through the parallel patterns in the crystal structure. This effect is even more pronounced when labradorite is polished.

Labradorite's mysterious blue sheen makes it a stone of magic, awakening awareness of different levels of energy all around us. In crystal healing, magic is understood to be an energy quality where things change, dissolve, or reform in surprising and unusual ways. Magic is strongly linked to intuition, that "gut feeling" or "sixth sense" that something is calling or communicating to you. Carrying or meditating with labradorite increases these shifts and twists of awareness. Labradorite is available in polished tumblestone form, set into jewelry, or carved into spheres and palm stones.

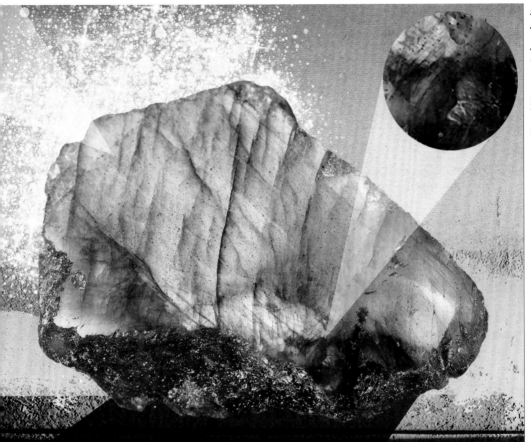

Opening the soul

In crystal healing, labradorite may be placed on the forehead, over the Third Eye Chakra, to open and stimulate awareness of magical energy. Placed over the top of the head, it can open the Crown Chakra to access information from higher energy levels. Labradorite is a crystal that suits those who want to explore different levels of energy, perception, and power. It is a symbol of the spiritual seeker and deepens your awareness of mystery and beauty.

Lapis Lazuli

Crystal facts

Hardness
5

Color
Vivid sapphire-blue with
tiny gold and white flecks

Geographical sources
Afghanistan, India, Myanmar,
Pakistan, Russia

Rarity
Fairly rare; source from
specialist suppliers

Form and structure
Forms within layers of rock
in the presence of many different
minerals, including lazarite

Chemical name
Sodium aluminum silicate with
sulfur, hydroxyl, and chlorine

Lapis lazuli literally means "blue stone," and is one of the most famous of all precious minerals. It was prized by the ancient Egyptians; the boy pharaoh Tutankhamun wore a gold collar in which lapis lazuli, carnelian, and onyx were set in pure gold. Because of its softness, lapis lazuli can be ground to a powder; the ancient Egyptians used it as eyeshadow. Medieval craftsmen melted powdered lapis lazuli into stained glass to make cathedral windows, such as in Chartres, France. The best-quality lapis lazuli is still found in Afghanistan, the oldest known source.

In crystal healing, lapis lazuli is linked to the Third Eye Chakra in the center of the forehead. This is the psychic center, the place of mystical visions. It is also in line with the location of the Uraeus, the sacred cobra depicted on the headdresses of the pharaohs, which symbolized divinity. Placing lapis lazuli on the forehead helps to open the Third Eye to receive spiritual guidance. It is also used for past-life journeying to connect to ancient wisdom you may hold.

Pointing the way

Lapis lazuli is a creative stone, a wonderful presence to keep with you if you need inspiration. Hold it, carry it, or meditate with it to increase your creativity and

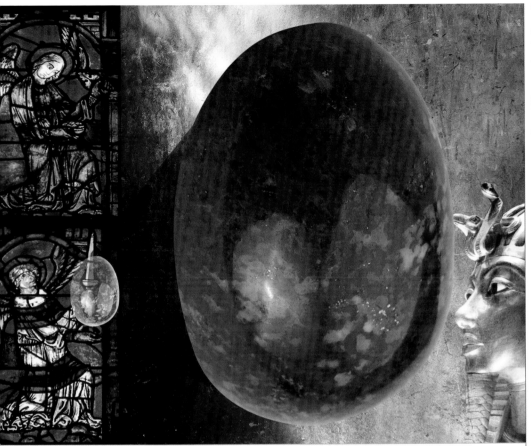

open your mind to new ideas. It helps you to maintain a "bird's eye view" of your life—an overview—which can help when your daily circumstances seem to bog you down. Lapis lazuli is like a shaft of light through clouds, illuminating your next step.

Buying lapis lazuli

Raw lapis pieces can be sourced from specialist suppliers. Polished lapis is usually available in the shape of spheres, eggs, hearts, or small carvings. It is the intensity of the blue color that shows the quality of a piece.

Merlinite

Crystal facts

Hardness
6–7

Color
An irregular mixture of gray, white, and black

Geographical sources
US

Rarity
Fairly rare; obtain from specialist suppliers

Form and structure
Forms in layered deposits, sometimes with tiny coatings of sparkling crystals called druzy

Chemical name
Silicon dioxide with manganese oxide

"Merlinite" is not the geological name of this crystal found in New Mexico, United States; it gained its name through its New Age use in crystal healing. It links to the magician Merlin, a key figure in the Arthurian legends, who had many magical powers, including the ability to shape-shift into different creatures. Merlinite is an unusual form of microcrystalline quartz fused with manganese oxide, which creates its irregular appearance; some areas are opaque and some are semitransparent. Hold a polished piece up to the light and you will see the interplay between the different layers.

Merlinite's irregular appearance has a moonlike quality that links it to the world of magic. It stimulates dreaming and enhances journeying during meditation, especially to different levels of energy or perception. Hold it or meditate with it to sharpen your intuition and increase your psychic awareness. When undertaking this journey, bear in mind that opening to inner levels of knowing is best done slowly; if you are unfamiliar with the ideas behind meditation journeys, try it out with the guidance of a crystal therapist.

Hearing yourself
In crystal healing, merlinite can be placed anywhere on the body where energy is blocked; it will help to dissolve the

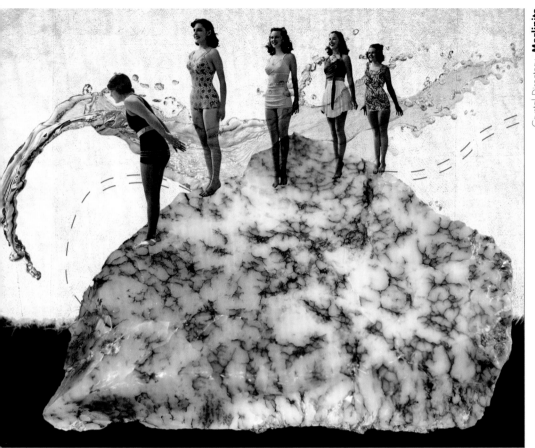

blockage and yield information about the cause. Investigating this can help you avoid such blocks in the future. Merlinite helps you to understand the messages that your energy body is trying to communicate to you; it opens pathways to inner wisdom. Merlinite also symbolizes the way energy is constantly changing from one state to another, helping you to "go with the flow."

Blue Lace Agate

Crystal facts

Hardness
7

Color
**Light blue, striped with bands
of pale and darker blue**

Geographical sources
South Africa, Brazil, Uruguay

Rarity
Widely available

Form and structure
Forms in large layered deposits

Chemical name
Silicon dioxide

The stripes and waves in blue lace agate identify it as part of the agate group of microcrystalline quartz. It is a beautiful crystal with delicate lines running through it, and when polished, it has a semitransparent appearance. It is often cut and polished into spheres or palm stones to hold; it is also shaped into beads, and the highest-quality pieces are set into jewelry. Small blue lace agate tumblestones are easily obtained. Blue lace agate is a popular choice when starting a crystal collection.

Blue lace agate has a gentle and cooling energy, working especially to ease the Throat Chakra and enable clear and honest communication. Because it clears the way for self-expression, it is a good crystal to carry for people who need to speak out but find this challenging to do.

Placed directly over the Throat Chakra, blue lace agate also soothes and cools sore throats, whether caused by too much speaking or illness.

The power of performance

It is a good stone to meditate with before, or carry during, public speaking, teaching, or making a presentation, as it focuses the energy of the Throat Chakra to make your

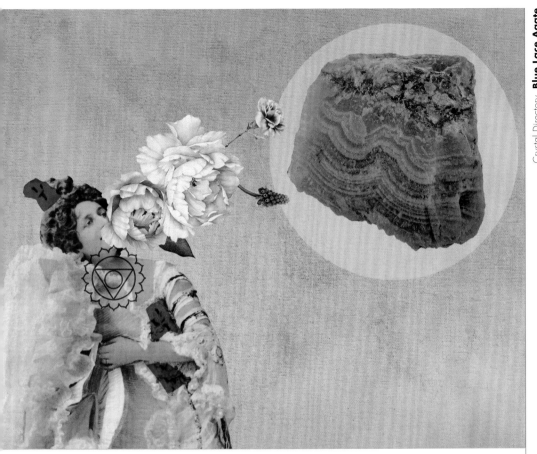

voice ring true. It is also useful for singers or performers to support voice projection. Meditation using sound, such as chanting mantras or other types of sacred music, is enhanced by holding blue lace agate. If you are working with affirmations, that is, saying positive intentions for your life out loud, then holding blue lace agate as you do this will enhance the energy of your words.

Resting easy

The gentle energy of blue lace agate makes it a great crystal to use with children. Placed in a child's bedroom it can help to create a calm atmosphere to help them sleep. It is also good for adults to hold or keep under the pillow for a restful night.

Chalcedony

Crystal facts

Hardness
7

Color
Vivid pale blue or pale lilac

Geographical sources
**Brazil, Czech Republic,
Madagascar, Mexico, India**

Rarity
Widely available

Form and structure
Forms in layered deposits

Chemical name
Silicon dioxide

Chalcedony is a type of layered microcrystalline quartz in which the microscopic crystals settle in swathes and lines through its surface. Chalcedony has a wonderful semitransparent appearance and a watery look; it may show inclusions (specks) of different minerals. Blue chalcedony is the most common; it is a very special shade of pale blue, with a hint of violet. Polished chalcedony has a beautiful shine and a soft silky feel when you touch it. It is widely available as polished tumblestones in various sizes.

Chalcedony is a soothing and calming crystal, useful in times of emotional and mental stress. It dissolves negative energy and allows it to flow away and out of the auric field. This is a good stone for people who tend to worry all the time, as it helps to calm obsessive thought patterns. Carrying chalcedony with you during the day can ease away stress and anxiety. You can also place a piece under your pillow at night to help release the baggage of the day and find peace and serenity in your sleep.

Speaking your truth
In crystal healing chalcedony is often placed over the Throat Chakra area to ease emotional or communication

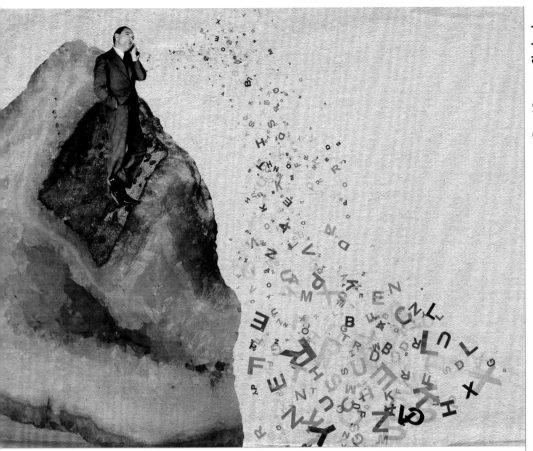

blockages in which the person is finding it hard to express their own truth. Chalcedony supports the healing of powerful inner feelings to allow clear words to be spoken. It also supports the voice in all ways—speaking, chanting, singing, performing—allowing the energy of the voice to flow with ease. Words are powerful: they can support or injure with ease. During times of emotional challenge, chalcedony acts as a soothing balm to clarify the messages you need to express.

Chrysocolla

Crystal facts

Hardness
2.5–3.5

Color
**Blue-green, deep green,
or turquoise**

Geographical sources
Russia, US, Africa

Rarity
Widely available

Form and structure
**Forms as massive amorphous
shapes, sometimes encrusted over
other rocks or in "grapelike" clusters**

Chemical name
Hydrated copper silicate

Chrysocolla is an unusual crystal with a fluid-looking, layered structure. The green color of chrysocolla is caused by the presence of copper silicate; it is often found alongside copper ore deposits with other blue-green stones like malachite (see pages 96–7). It is very soft and breaks or scratches easily, so store it with care.

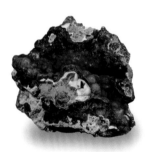

The vivid blue-green mottled color of chrysocolla reminds us of the image of the Earth taken from the moon: a beautiful swirling turquoise disk. The energy of the chrysocolla crystal connects us to nature and the Earth in a vibrant way through the Heart Chakra; it teaches us to love and appreciate the planet that we inhabit. Meditating with it creates an intuitive connection with the earth.

Creative empowerment

The combination of shades within chrysocolla link the Heart Chakra (green) to the Throat Chakra (blue). Chrysocolla supports the expression of feeling from the heart in positive and creative ways through speaking, singing, artistic creation, performing, and opening up to full self-expression. It is a particularly useful crystal for singers to carry, as it

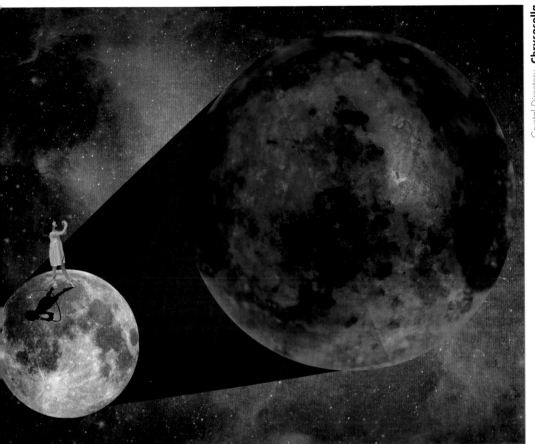

stimulates the voice to convey the energy of love. It is also a good crystal to carry with you if communication issues occur in your work, as it supports clear and positive energy through your voice.

Bringing back health

Chrysocolla also promotes life force and physical vitality; it helps to restore the body after long periods of illness. Holding chrysocolla or placing a piece under the pillow helps to encourage replenishing sleep, which is the body's best way to recover. In crystal healing it is often placed over the Heart Chakra or the Solar Plexus Chakra (just under the rib cage) to restore depleted energy.

Sapphire

Crystal facts

Hardness
9

Color
**Mostly deep blue; also pink,
white and yellow types**

Geographical sources
**Australia, Afghanistan, India,
Myanmar, Pakistan, Sri Lanka**

Rarity
**Gem-quality stones are rare;
lower-grade granular pieces are
widely available**

Form and structure
**Forms as six-sided crystals, with
prismatic or rhombohedral shapes**

Chemical name
Aluminum oxide

Sapphires have a similar story to rubies (see pages 112–3). They also form beautiful six-sided gems, which are faceted and polished to show a glorious deep blue color thanks to the presence of titanium and iron in the aluminum oxide. Though blue is the most common color associated with sapphire, it also occurs in other colors such as pink and yellow. As well as high-grade, gem-quality crystal deposits used to make jewelry, sapphire also forms in granular layers, and pieces of this lower-grade crystal are widely available through crystal suppliers.

Blue sapphire is a stone of great tranquility; it cools and soothes the mind, linking to the Third Eye Chakra in the center of the forehead. Even if you do not possess a gem-quality blue sapphire, if you visualize one in the middle of your forehead as you meditate, you will feel the gentle cooling quality of sapphire energy in your mind. It encourages mental focus and clarity, helping to bring order to scattered thoughts.

This is a stone traditionally associated with wisdom, a calm sense of inner knowing. Carry or wear blue sapphire to feel a quiet sense of self-confidence; it helps you find the right words and the right ways to be in situations that confront you.

Calm clarity

In crystal layouts, blue sapphire can be placed over the Third Eye Chakra or the

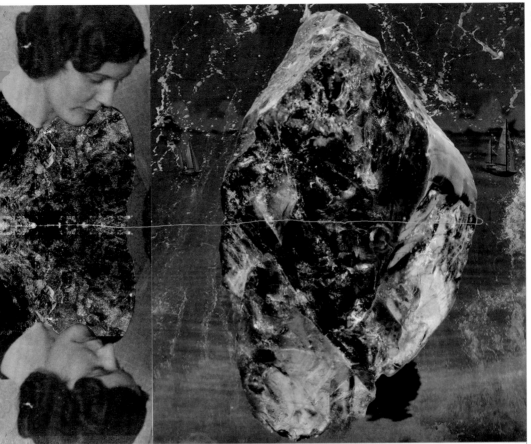

Throat Chakra to encourage inner
wisdom and calm communication. If a
person's emotions are highly inflamed,
placing a piece of blue sapphire over the
Heart Chakra in the center of the chest
helps to soothe overstimulated feelings.

Calcite

Crystal facts

Hardness
3

Colors
**Clear, honey-colored,
pink, green, orange, blue**

Geographical sources
Mexico, South Africa, US

Rarity
**Widely available in opaque colors;
clear and semitransparent variations
are less common**

Form and structure
**Forms in chunks, stalactites,
or layered deposits**

Chemical name
Calcium carbonate

Calcite is the crystalized form of calcium carbonate, also known as limestone; this is a mineral that makes up about 5 percent of the Earth's surface. Limestone formed millions of years ago through the breakdown of shells of sea creatures falling and settling into rocky layers at the bottom of ancient oceans. As the tectonic plates of the Earth squeezed and shifted against each other, the ancient ocean beds were lifted up to form mountain ranges; even the Himalayas are made of limestone. Calcite formations are incredibly varied and abundant and are found all over the world.

Clear calcite

Clear calcite is also called Iceland spar. It looks like glass and has the ability to double-refract light, so if you look through it, everything appears twice. It is a crystal used to promote inner vision and spiritual awakening, and awareness that there are always other layers of perception available. Clear calcite can be placed anywhere on the body to cleanse and shift blocked energy. It restores and regenerates the entire auric field.

Honey calcite

Pale golden honey calcite works particularly with the Solar Plexus Chakra (just under the middle of the rib cage), where it supports this chakra's highest spiritual function, encouraging personal power and energy to work to their most

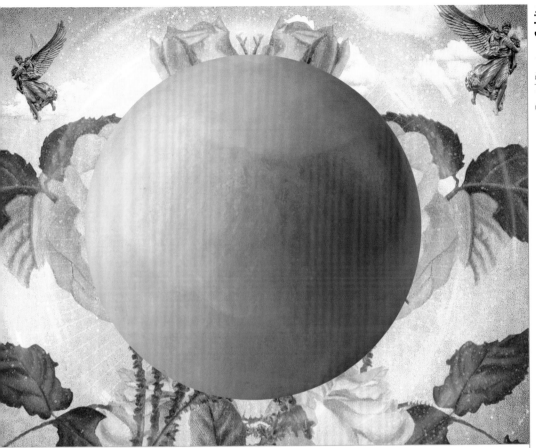

noble purpose. As a golden crystal, honey calcite also attracts abundance; carry it or place it in the northwest corner of your home, which is associated with prosperity.

rose quartz. It opens the Heart Chakra to receive unconditional love. Hold or carry pink calcite during times of emotional stress to feel supported and nurtured.

Pink calcite

Pink calcite can be found in opaque and transparent forms; its energy is similar to

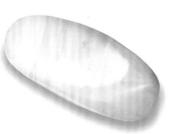

Calcite crystals can be found in a wide variety of colors, the most striking of which come from Mexico. Calcite crystal formations tend to be made up of geometric shapes and angles; they also display defined vertical striations or perfect vertical planes. The stones are usually opaque but rare semitransparent or clear pieces can be obtained.

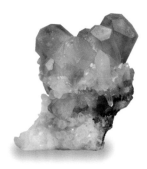

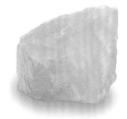

Green calcite

This type of calcite is a gentle pale green in color, though some rarer pieces carry a deeper shade. It is a refreshing crystal to hold or carry; it clears blocked emotional energy, bringing a general sense of balance and well-being. In crystal healing it can be placed directly over the Heart Chakra in an emotionally cleansing layout, to help release old emotional burdens and bring a feeling of lightness and inner peace.

Orange calcite

This calcite varies between pale orange to vibrant tangerine in color. It has a cheering energy and encourages a positive approach to change. It resonates with the Sacral Chakra, helping to encourage creativity in all forms and

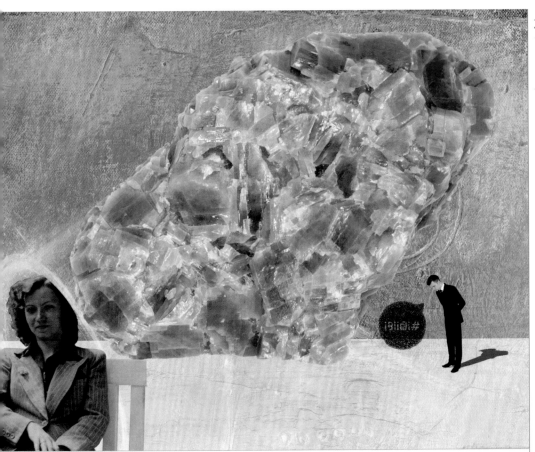

transforming lethargy into revitalized purpose. Larger pieces radiate positive energy, particularly when positioned in the center of your home, which is the place of health and balance in Feng Shui.

Blue calcite

This is a beautiful variety of calcite with a soft blue radiance. Some higher-quality pieces have a liquid look to them, like water held frozen in time. In crystal healing, blue calcite envelops the aura in gentle healing light, protecting it from other people's invasive thoughts, emotions, and words. Placed over the Throat Chakra it cools physical or emotional inflammation; over the Third Eye in the center of the forehead, it calms emotional stress and soothes headaches.

Jade

Crystal facts

Hardness
6.5–7

Color
Pale or vivid green,
cream, red, black, with rare
purple or blue forms

Geographical sources
Nephrite: Canada, India, New
Zealand, US; jadeite: Myanmar,
Russia, Japan

Rarity
Widely available, though cost
varies greatly

Form and structure
Microcrystalline layers

Chemical names
Nephrite: calcium magnesium
silicate; jadeite: sodium aluminum
silicate (both are traded as jade)

The story of jade is one of two minerals. Nephrite tends to be a pale green or cream color; jadeite is a deeper green, red, black, or even blue shade. In the nineteenth century, mineralogical techniques enabled these two minerals to be distinguished from each other; until that time they had both been called jade, and today they are still both sold under that name. In China, jade has always been a most venerated and precious mineral, often carved into priceless jade statues. Today, simple jade pieces, polished spheres, or tumblestones are available at reasonable prices.

In crystal healing, nephrite and jadeite are considered together as jade, with healing properties according to the color variations. The following are the most common types.

Green jade

Green jade can vary from pale green to vivid shades. It is a Heart Chakra stone, symbolizing the abundance of nature;

it stimulates true prosperity in life. Placing a green jade sphere or a Laughing Buddha in the Feng Shui wealth and prosperity area of your home (northwest corner) helps to increase the flow of abundance to you.

Red jade

Deep red jade symbolizes courage and protection; carry it when you need to put aside worry or fear and do what has to

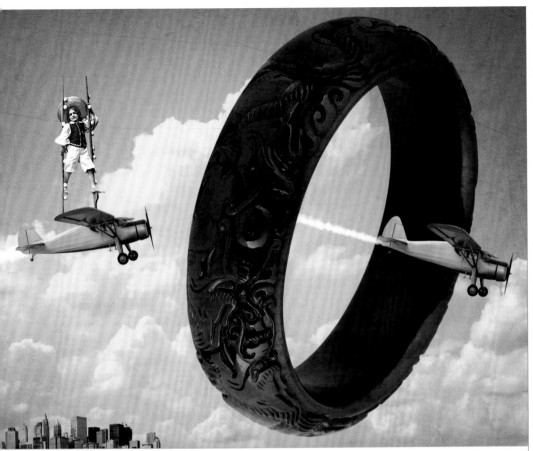

be done. Red jade links to the Root Chakra at the base of the spine; it grounds and warms the physical body and gives it the energy to take action. This gem promotes physical strength, passion, and vitality.

Black jade

Black jade acts like a shield, protecting you from negative influences of any kind, whether from people, places, or electromagnetic stress. It is an extremely beneficial stone to carry whenever you travel, as it diverts negativity back into the Earth, away from your auric field and neutralized.

Moonstone

Crystal facts

Hardness
7

Color
Varies

Geographical sources
**Sri Lanka, India, Myanmar,
Australia, India, US**

Rarity
Widely available

Form and structure
**Forms as blocks or
prismatic structures, often
with granite**

Chemical name
Potassium aluminum silicate

Moonstone is one of the most popular crystals in New Age and spiritual healing. Its gentle radiance is due to an effect called labradorescence, where light rays bounce back and forth within hairlike layers inside the crystal structure, creating a special sheen as the stone is turned toward a light source. Moonstone is very popular set in silver and worn as jewelry. Different kinds of moonstone have varied color and sheen effects; the most popular are shown here and on the next pages. Raw pieces, polished palm stones, or tumblestones are available for use in crystal healing.

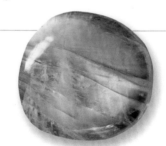

Blue moonstone

This kind of moonstone has a pale blue color, and its sheen is a vivid blue as it is turned to the light. It is a stone of the Goddess, symbolizing sacred feminine energy; it enhances awareness of the moon and all its cycles. People frequently wear it to balance the hormones and calm emotional or nervous stress: it is a very gentle crystal and has a soothing vibration.

In crystal healing, blue moonstone can be placed over the Sacral Chakra (below the navel) or on the Root Chakra area (base of the spine) to help balance and restore the reproductive organs.

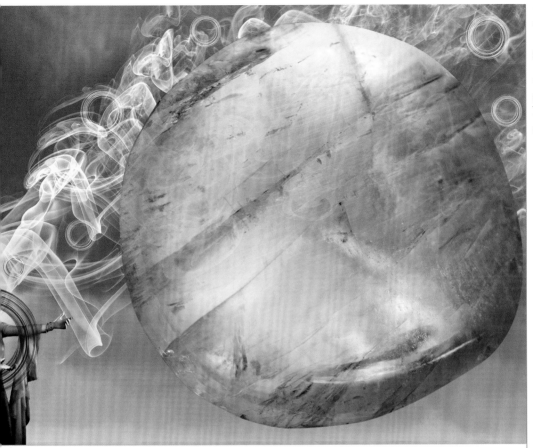

Rainbow moonstone

This variety of moonstone shows shimmering blue, green, and gold shades as it is turned to the light. It is more powerful than blue moonstone, enhancing psychic awareness and intuition and working to open the Third Eye Chakra in the center of the forehead. Its shimmering colors open the mind to endless new possibilities, stimulating imaginative thinking and artistic creativity. Wearing rainbow moonstone attracts positive energy into your life and improves your self-confidence.

Moonstone has been valued for centuries as a mystical crystal with the power to balance the emotions. Just because it is strongly linked to feminine energy this does not mean it is only for women; men can also benefit from its soothing and mysterious lunar radiance. For men, any type of moonstone encourages the mind to be receptive, to slow down and listen to inner guidance. The color of moonstone you are drawn to is the right one for your energy at this time.

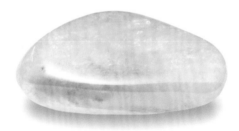

White moonstone

This type of moonstone is the one that looks most like the full moon itself; it shimmers with a luminous white radiance. When the moon is full, it is reflecting the light of the sun; the two are in complete harmony. Full moon is a time of psychic perception where dreams can be particularly clear or meaningful. Meditating with white moonstone at the full moon, or wearing this stone at this time, will allow you to experience lunar energy at its most powerful. In crystal healing, white moonstone can be placed over the Third Eye Chakra in the center of the forehead to stimulate heightened perception of dreams. Placed over the Heart Chakra in the center of the chest, white moonstone also balances and soothes the emotions, bringing inner peace and tranquility.

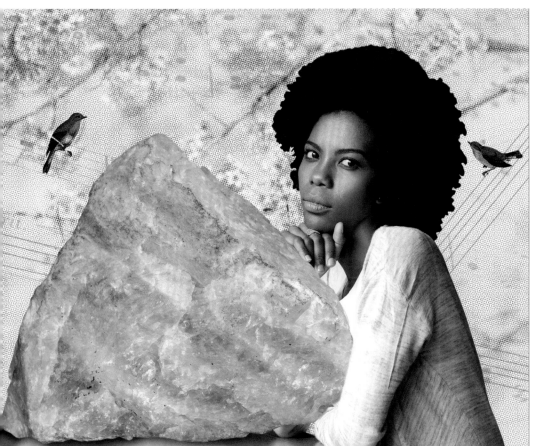

Peach moonstone

This type of moonstone is a rarer variation and tends to be more costly. The background color is a soft peach or pale orange color; the sheen is pale blue and violet. It is a very gentle form of moonstone with an extremely soothing effect on delicate emotions, calming worry and emotional stress, and bringing a sense of inner balance. It is a very helpful form of moonstone to use with adults or children who are highly anxious and stressed by their environment.

Jasper

Crystal facts

Hardness
6.5

Color
Mostly red, brown, yellow; many
multicolored types exist

Geographical sources
All over the world, especially
Brazil, India, France, Germany,
US, Australia

Rarity
Widely available

Form and structure
Forms in layered deposits,
nodules, or fillings in fissures
in rock layers

Chemical name
Silicon dioxide

Jasper is a very common mineral found all over the world in different colors, including many multicolored varieties, which vary according to the different mineral composition of surrounding rocks. It is an opaque form of microcrystalline quartz, polishing up to a silken sheen. It is often available as carved heart shapes, spheres, statues, or as simple polished tumblestones. Here we look at the most common colored varieties.

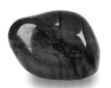

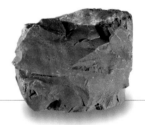

Red jasper

This type of jasper has been valued for centuries as a protective and strengthening stone. It stimulates vitality and life energy and works to enhance the Root Chakra at the base of the spine. It is good to carry when feeling low, weak, or lacking in physical strength. It also enhances personal presence and helps to build confidence in social situations.

Brown jasper

Brown jasper stimulates Earth energy, connecting to qualities of deep peace, stability, and protection. It shields the entire aura from negative electromagnetic or environmental stress. It is a good stone to place by the front door as a guardian of your home. In healing layouts, brown jasper can be placed between the feet for a grounding and stabilizing effect.

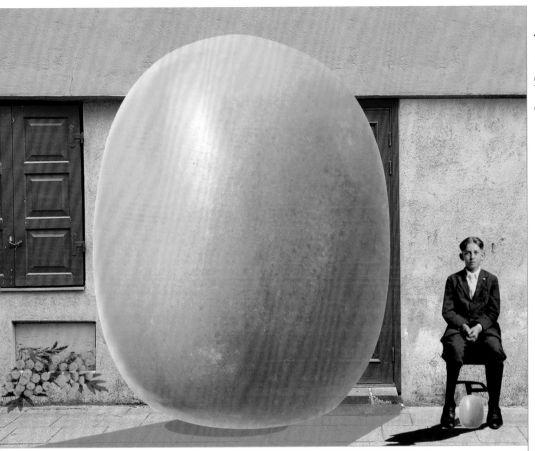

Yellow jasper

This variety of jasper links to the Solar Plexus Chakra; it builds self-confidence and supports clear decision-making. It also eases digestive problems linked to emotional stress. Placed in a living room, pieces of yellow jasper help to clear negative energies from your space.

Multicolored jasper

Different multicolored varieties of jasper keep appearing on the market; a recent example is mookaite, a red Australian jasper with beautiful cream and gold patterns. In crystal therapy mookaite is used to support ancestral healing, releasing old energy patterns from a family's past.

Tourmaline

Crystal facts

Hardness
7–7.5

Color
**Black, pink, "watermelon"
(green and pink)**

Geographical sources
Brazil, US, Pakistan, Nepal

Rarity
**Fairly rare; obtain from
specialist crystal suppliers**

Form and structure
**Forms as distinctive vertical
columns with striations**

Chemical name
**Aluminum borosilicate
hydroxide oxide**

Tourmalines are a family of crystals that have become very popular since the nineteenth century. They have vertical shapes and striations (lines) running down the sides of their structure. They are very popular in crystal healing, and all three varieties have particular energetic uses. Tourmaline crystals are rare and expensive to buy; their structure does not lend itself to polishing, so raw pieces will tend to be available. Fine tourmaline pieces are also valued by mineralogist collectors, so this limits the commercial availability of these crystals.

Black tourmaline

Also known as schorl, this distinctive black crystal has strong protective and detoxifying energy. Wearing or carrying black tourmaline is a good idea if your work or travel takes you into challenging situations: the crystal works like an energy shield, keeping negative or intrusive energy at bay. Black tourmaline has a channeling quality due to the vertical nature of its structure; it helps negativity or blocked energy to move on and out of the auric field. This is a crystal that benefits from being buried in the ground from time to time to allow its energy to be neutralized by the Earth, so the crystal is recharged and ready for use.

In crystal healing, black tourmaline is often placed between or under the feet to add its protective channeling power

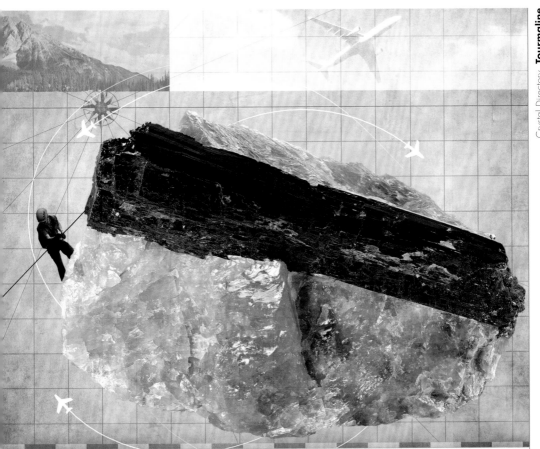

to healing layouts. It also helps to cleanse
and purify the energy field of the person
being treated.

Tourmalines are known for a particular effect called piezoelectricity, which means that if the crystal is heated or rubbed, a different electrical charge will occur at each end of the crystal. Tourmalines are active channelers and movers of energy; they attract and move it through and onward. This is why they are valued so much in crystal healing.

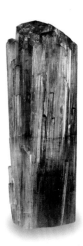

Watermelon tourmaline

This unusual form of tourmaline unites a deep pink color with a rich green shade. Sometimes columns of watermelon tourmaline form with a green outer layer and a pink inner layer, or long blades form with a balance between the two colors. This form of tourmaline unites both colors that are associated with the Heart Chakra: green for growth, expansion, and feelings of love for other people, and pink for unconditional and spiritual love for all beings. Watermelon tourmaline reminds us that love takes many forms, and that balancing the human with the spiritual is the best harmony of all.

Pink tourmaline

This variety of tourmaline varies in color from the palest pink to the deepest rose.

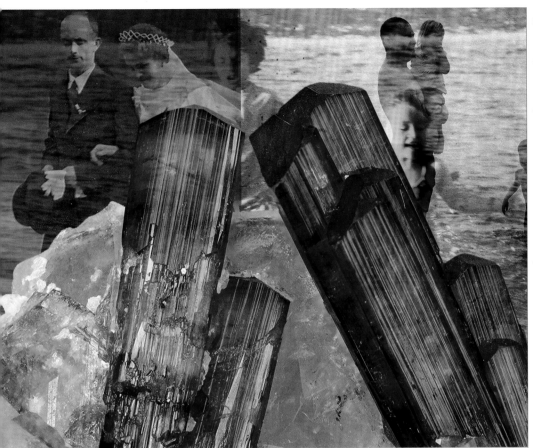

Its transparency also varies; the best-quality pieces have a beautiful watery appearance. Pink tourmaline is hugely valued as a Heart Chakra activator; it opens the heart to give and receive love. Because of the channeling aspect of tourmaline, this crystal works particularly well to free up the emotions of people who are closed off or under great stress. It also helps with recovery from grief, helping to move through feelings and feel more hopeful again. Pink tourmaline brings a renewed zest for life and a sense of vitality and spontaneity. Wear or carry pink tourmaline to stay open to all the positive energy that wants to enter your life. Meditate with pink tourmaline to send out love to your friends, family, and the wider world.

Topaz

Crystal facts

Hardness
8

Color
Blue, white, or golden

Geographical sources
Brazil, Sri Lanka, Myanmar,
Australia, Japan, Mexico,
Masagascar

Rarity
Rare; obtain from specialist
crystal suppliers

Form and structure
Forms as eight-sided
prismatic crystals with striations
(lines) along the main axis

Chemical name
Aluminum silicate fluoride
hydroxide

Topaz is a precious stone that can be cut, faceted, and polished because of its hardness. Top-quality gems are reserved for fine jewelry making, but lower-grade specimens are sometimes available through crystal suppliers. Colorless topaz can be irradiated to create artificial and different colors; true natural shades are blue, white, or golden (sometimes called imperial topaz). For crystal healing purposes it is always best to work with natural stones because these are a true reflection of Earth energy.

Blue topaz

This variety of topaz is a very gentle pale blue crystal with a quiet and calming effect on the Throat Chakra, where it soothes fiery emotions and encourages positive communication. Placed over the Third Eye Chakra in the middle of the forehead, blue topaz calms the mind and encourages clear thinking, which is especially good for people whose minds are scattered and distracted. Blue topaz also enables a gentle opening of the Third Eye Chakra, which is beneficial to anyone beginning their own spiritual journey. It encourages a steady expansion and exploration of higher energy levels.

White (clear) topaz

Clear topaz is a stone of manifestation; it holds and reflects the vibration of energy

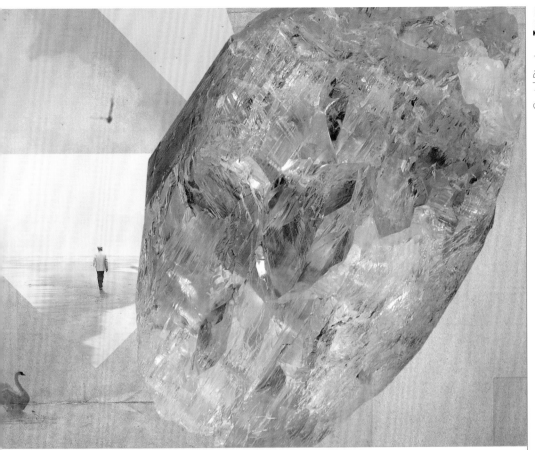

that is put into it. If you want positive results, think positive thoughts when you are holding it. Clear topaz helps you to focus your intentions. It is good to work with it when you are planning a new project or a new direction in your life. It is an extremely creative crystal and can be placed anywhere on the body to dissolve blocked energy and revitalize the auric field.

Golden topaz

Golden topaz links to the Solar Plexus Chakra in the upper abdomen; its color reflects solar light and brilliance, increasing vitality and physical energy. It is an abundance attractor, so place a piece in the Feng Shui wealth area in the northwest corner of your home.

Obsidian

Crystal facts

Hardness
5.5

Color
**Black, black with
white specks, or black with
rainbow iridescence**

Geographical sources
US, Italy, Mexico, Britain

Rarity
Widely available

Form and structure
**Forms as amorphous
volcanic glass**

Chemical name
Silicon dioxide

Obsidian is a kind of glass, fused in the heat of volcanic activity; it originally formed along the edges of lava flows where water was present. Human beings have been fascinated with this crystal since prehistoric times. In southern parts of the United States, thousands of ancient arrowheads have been found, carefully shaped from slivers of obsidian, which makes razor-sharp edges. Obsidian was a favorite tool of the ancient world. It was also a stone of magic, carried by medicine men as an energy shield and a badge of power.

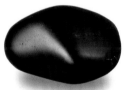

There are different types of obsidian; on this and the next pages we will look at three of the most common and important forms for crystal healing.

Black obsidian

This is the most common form of obsidian. It is available as raw chunks, or as smooth, polished palm stones, or tumblestones. It has a dense, glossy black color; some pieces show waves or curving lines that formed as the crystal cooled. You may also find raw pieces with very sharp edges.

Black obsidian offers powerful psychic protection to ward off negative energies and acts as a shield against environmental stress. Placing a piece under the bed at night offers protection from bad dreams; carrying a piece gives protection from

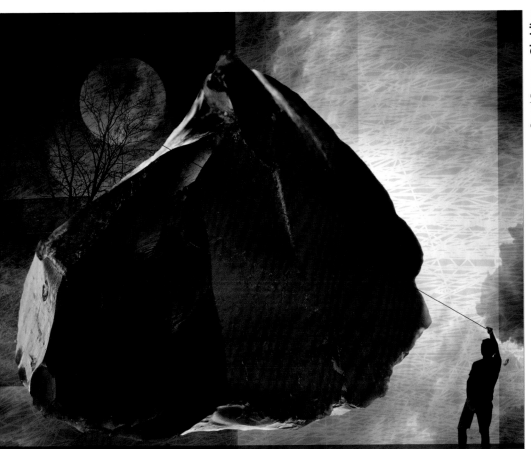

negative energies as you go about your day. Meditate with black obsidian to cleanse any negativity from your aura, sensing the crystal dissolving and absorbing any negative thought patterns or emotions. Occasionally, it is beneficial to bury your piece of obsidian in soil and leave it overnight to allow the Earth's energy to cleanse it and neutralize any negativity it has absorbed.

In crystal healing, black obsidian is often placed between or under the feet to channel any negative energy out of the auric field. Black obsidian grounds any crystal layout, providing a protective shield during guided meditation journeys.

Obsidian comes in different varieties, each with particular healing qualities. It is worth noting that in recent times, pale blue and pale green "obsidian" varieties have appeared on the market; though these are pretty to look at, they are in fact just manufactured glass. True obsidian has deep, dense dark colors and an aura of mystery about it.

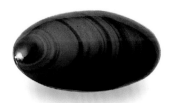

Rainbow obsidian

This is an unusual and rarer form of obsidian in which, at a particular angle, the stone will show a sheen of red, blue, green, and gold colors. Rainbow obsidian pieces are usually cut and polished to enhance this effect. It is a beautifully mysterious crystal because it looks black and opaque at some angles, and then transforms in the presence of light.

In crystal healing, rainbow obsidian helps to transform all negative energies and influences and brings them into the light of healing. It has a positive cleansing effect on all seven chakras. However tired or depleted the person being treated may be, rainbow obsidian helps to lift them. In a crystal layout, it can be placed anywhere on the body where energy needs restoring.

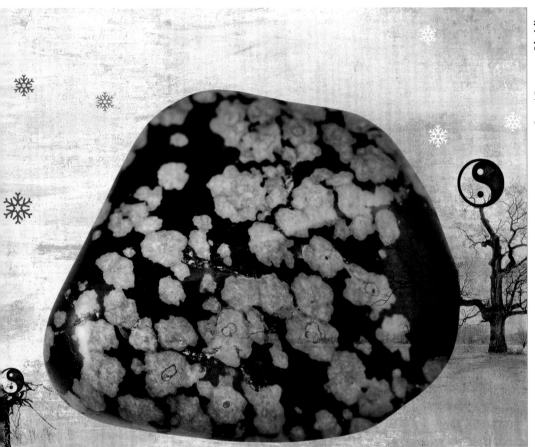

Snowflake obsidian

This is a variety of obsidian in which the volcanic glass is spotted with small, snowflake-shaped white specks, which appeared as the crystal formed. The contrast of black and white shows that dark and light, positive and negative, or yin/yang energies are always present and it is important to find balance. This is a good stone to carry to remind yourself that you have the power to find balance in your own life, whatever the outside world is telling you. Snowflake obsidian has a similar protective effect to black obsidian, but is considered to have a gentler intensity. In healing layouts, it is often placed over the Solar Plexus Chakra, where it restores a positive sense of personal power and balances body, mind, and spirit.

Fluorite

Crystal facts

Hardness
4

Colors
Pale to deep purple; purple, pink,
and green striped; rich green

Geographical sources
Brazil, Canada, China, US,
Britain, Argentina

Rarity
Widely available in all colors

Form and structure
Forms in cubic or octahedral
crystals, with clear geometric lines

Chemical name
Calcium fluoride

Fluorite forms in hydrothermal veins within rock layers; it is often found alongside quartz and calcite. It is called fluorite because it glows under ultraviolet light, showing an effect called fluorescence. Fluorite is also thermoluminescent, meaning that it glows brightly if it is heated. It is a very common mineral compound, found in many countries around the world. Structurally, it is very orderly; if pieces are struck in the correct way, it is easy to create perfect octahedral shapes. Many of the lower-grade, less expensive pieces of fluorite on sale have been shaped like this.

The geometric structure of fluorite gives it healing properties linked to form, stability, and a state of balance. It brings coherence and perspective to the mind; if placed over the Third Eye Chakra in the middle of the forehead, or over the Crown Chakra at the top of the head, this can resolve muddled thinking and improve perception.

Purple fluorite
This is the most common color variation of fluorite. The shade is a beautiful, semitranslucent lavender purple, which becomes even more vivid when the stone is polished. The intensity of the color varies; choose what feels right to you.

Purple fluorite is an excellent crystal to have with you in the workplace or when

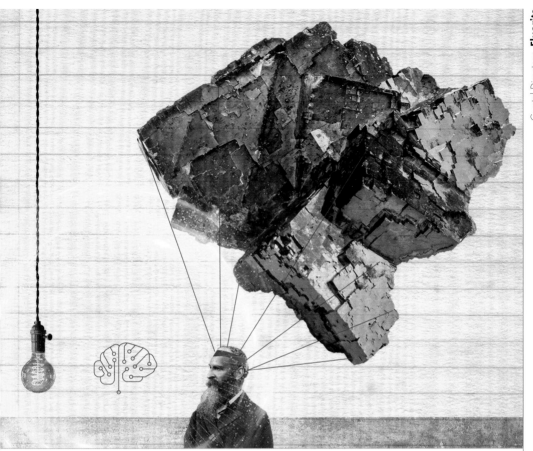

studying to keep your head clear and assist with tasks that require focus and concentration. It calms anxiety and feelings of overload and helps to find solutions to puzzles and challenges.

Fluorite can be found in many different colors, but the variations below are two of the most useful fluorite crystals from a healing perspective. The overall meaning of fluorite is achieving balance and a clear mind, finding structure and space instead of feeling confused. Fluorite in general helps to focus the mind and spirit, and these two color variations have their own particular healing vibrations.

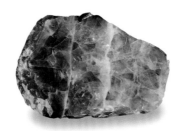

Rainbow fluorite

This beautiful crystal shows bands of purple and green through its structure. Every piece is unique because the patterns are so varied. Rainbow fluorite is even more stunning when it is polished, where the play of colors can be fully appreciated. The best-quality pieces are used to make jewelry. Although rainbow fluorite is more expensive than the purple variety, the range of pieces available offers something for everyone.

The colors in rainbow fluorite symbolize a link between the Crown Chakra (purple) and the Heart Chakra (green). The Crown Chakra is the energy center where spiritual expansion occurs; the Heart Chakra's energy is of growth and the expression of compassion for all beings. A link between these two chakras allows

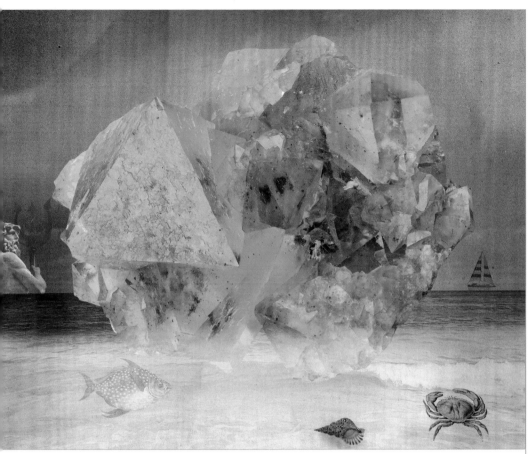

spiritual energy to enter the heart, and the heart to expand into a wider awareness of divine love. Placing a piece of rainbow fluorite over the Heart Chakra or holding a piece in each hand helps to create this link between heart and spirit.

Green fluorite

Pure green fluorite is a rare form of fluorite with a particularly vivid green color. It looks like sea water frozen in time. Meditating with a piece of green fluorite connects you to the vibration of the sea and its creatures, and to the ancient mythical sea-kingdom of Atlantis. The lines and angles within green fluorite look like ancient temples or structures. Green fluorite opens your heart to the energy of the blue-green water mantle of the Earth.

Tiger's Eye

Crystal facts

Hardness
7

Color
Golden yellow, red, or blue

Geographical sources
**South Africa, India,
Myanmar, Australia, US**

Rarity
Widely available

Form and structure
**Forms as fibrous
massed deposits**

Chemical name
Silicon dioxide

Tiger's eye is a kind of microcrystalline quartz that forms in layers with fibrous strands which reflect the light back at each other to create a shimmering effect called chatoyancy. The most common type is golden yellow. Some deposits in South Africa have a reddish color, though pieces of true red tiger's eye are rare and many sold with that label have been dyed. A blue variety of tiger's eye also comes from South Africa. Tiger's eye is one of the most popular crystals in a starter collection.

Yellow tiger's eye

This variety is a stone of vitality, strength, and inner harmony. Its golden sheen links it to the Solar Plexus Chakra just under the middle of the rib cage; this is the "solar center" of the body and it responds to yellow tiger's eye by opening and re-energizing itself. Yellow tiger's eye is also a stone of abundance; place a large piece in the Feng Shui wealth area of your living space (the northwest corner) to encourage a rich flow into your life. Carry or wear yellow tiger's eye to protect you from any negative energy during the day.

Red tiger's eye

This is a warming stone for Root Chakra energy; placed on the base of the spine, it encourages the body to feel energized and strengthened. It is a good stone

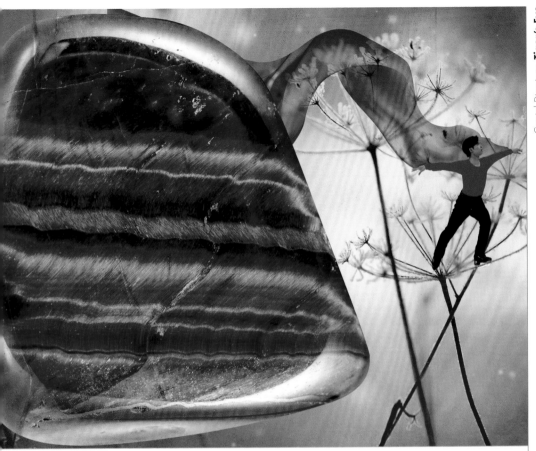

to wear or carry in the wintertime when the body's energy is colder and weaker. Red tiger's eye also stimulates Root Chakra reproductive energy in both men and women.

Blue tiger's eye (hawk's eye)

Mysterious blue tiger's eye is sometimes called hawk's eye because it looks more like the eye of a bird. It resonates with the Throat Chakra (communication) and the Third Eye Chakra (inspiration), helping to stimulate creative expression. In crystal layouts it is often placed in the center of the forehead to enhance inner vision and a higher understanding of life situations.

Metals

Crystal facts

Hardness
Gold: 2–3. Silver: 2–3. Copper: 3

Color
Gold: yellow
Silver: whitish-gray
Copper: orange-yellow

Geographical sources
Gold: South Africa, US
Silver: Mexico, Canada
Copper: Australia, US

Rarity
All these metals are rare ores

Form and structure
All form as metallic ores
within rock layers

Chemical names
Gold (element symbol: Au)
Silver (element symbol: Ag)
Copper (element symbol: Cu)

The three metals considered here are the three most commonly associated with healing. They are sometimes available as nuggets in the case of gold or silver, or as pieces of pure copper ore; you may find these if you look around crystal fairs or visit specialist crystal or mineral suppliers. Most often precious metals will be incorporated into jewelry or into crystal healing tools such as wands with different crystals fused together; silver or copper often feature here. Gold is, of course, one of the rarest of all metals, and will most likely feature as a setting for a gem or stone.

Gold

Pure gold symbolizes the radiance and intense light of the sun. It has a long association with power and majesty. Its radiance links with the Solar Plexus Chakra, where it cleanses and clears blocked energy and restores vitality. Visualizing the gold energy ray is a technique often used in healing to clear stagnation and return the aura to its full potency. Wearing crystals set in gold helps to harmonize and regulate the body's own energy field.

Silver

Silver is associated with the cool, soft light of the moon. It is a favorite setting for crystal healing jewelry. Silver soothes and calms the body and mind; it has a gently

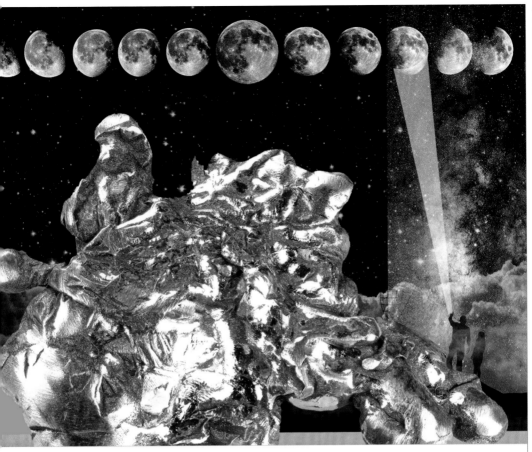

harmonizing effect on the subtle systems of the body, such as the hormones or the immune system. Silver also encourages intuitive connection with the lunar cycles, from new to waxing to full to waning. It helps you stay aware and balanced during times of change.

Copper

Orange-tinged copper is a metal that conducts electricity, and acts as a strong energy channel. Crystal wands wound with copper wire and smaller stones set in copper make powerful tools for experienced crystal healers to use in treatments. These wands help to direct energy through and around the body for healing purposes.

215

GLOSSARY

Agate
A type of quartz with a microcrystalline structure and distinctive bands.

Aggregate
A basic rock composed of coarse- to medium-grained types of sand.

Amorphous
A mineral with no internal structure and an irregular shape, such as obsidian.

Aura
A term describing the energetic field that extends around the physical human body. Healing methods, including crystal healing, aim to rebalance and revitalize the aura; when the energy field is strong again, the physical body is restored and the mind is calm.

Cabochon
A shaped crystal with a flat base and polished dome surface.

Chakra
A term describing an energy center in the body (from the Sanskrit for "wheel").

Chatoyancy
A light effect named from the French phrase *œil de chat*, meaning cat's eye.

Cleavage
The angle in a crystal along which it will split.

Columnar
Tall, thin crystals shaped like columns.

Cubic
In the form of a cube, a three-dimensional, four-sided structure.

Dichroic
A mineral that shows different colors when held at different angles, such as tourmaline.

Encrustation
A mass of tiny crystals that forms as a crust over a base rock layer.

Facet
Angled crystal face, either natural (quartz) or man-made (cut ruby).

Feldspar
A large group of common minerals formed of aluminum silicate.

Geode
Geodes start out as bubbles in volcanic rock; over millions of years, the outer layers harden. Mineral-rich water seeps through causing crystals to form inside the cavity.

Igneous
A rock produced by fire or volcanic activity.

Inclusion
A mineral contained within another crystal, for example rutile strands in rutilated quartz.

Inorganic
Naturally occurring chemical compounds that are not living.

Iridescence
A play of rainbow colors, such as rainbow moonstone.

Labradorescence
A shimmering effect of contrasting color, such as labradorite.

Mineral
A naturally occurring solid chemical compound, such as silicon dioxide (quartz).

Mineraloid
A mineral that does not display crystalline geometry, such as amorphous volcanic glass (obsidian), molten meteorite glass (tektite or moldavite), or jet (compacted coal).

Opalescence
A rippling sheen of rainbow hues, such as is seen in opal.

Organic
If the word is used in a mineral sense, it means a compound originally from a living source, for example, amber, which originally occurred as resin from pine trees before it became fossilized.

Piezoelectric
A crystal that carries an electrical charge after rubbing or striking, for example, all types of quartz and topaz.

Pleochroism
Ripples of different colors depending on the angle of light, such as kunzite or tanzanite.

Refraction
Light diverted to a different angle due to a crystal's geometric structure.

Rock (or stone)
A natural substance, a solid combination of one or more minerals or mineraloids. For example, granite, a common rock, is a combination of the minerals quartz, feldspar, and biotite.

Striations
Natural grooves along a crystal's surface.

Tabular
A term that describes crystals shaped like slabs.

Tectonic plates
Sections of the Earth's crust that float on the inner mantle and constantly move, very slowly, over millions of years.

Tektite
Crystals formed when meteorites hit the earth and melt silica (sand) deposits on the surface, creating a molten glass structure, such as moldavite.

Termination
A pointed crystal tip, for example, clear quartz.

FURTHER READING

Ahsian, Naisha, *The Crystal Ally Cards*, Crystalis Institute Press, 2017

Frazier, Karen, *Crystals for Healing*, Althea Press, 2015

Hall, Judy, *The Crystal Bible Vols 1, 2, 3*, Godsfield Press, 2009

Harding, Jennie, *Crystals*, Chartwell Books, 2016

Lilly, Simon and Sue Lilly *Crystal Healing: The Practical Guide To Using Crystals For Health And Well-Being*, Watkins, 2010

Park, Graham, *Introducing Geology*, Dunedin Academic Press, 2010

Rothery, David, *Geology: A Complete Introduction*, Teach Yourself, 2016

Silbey, Uma, *The Ultimate Guide to Crystals and Stones*, Skyhorse Publishing, 2016

Simmons, Robert and Ahsian, Naisha, *The Book of Stones*, 2nd edn., North Atlantic Books, 2015

USEFUL ADDRESSES & WEBSITES

Contact these organizations if you are interested in training as a crystal healer or seeking a qualified therapist in your area.

US CRYSTAL HEALING ASSOCIATIONS

The Association of Melody Crystal Healers International
info@melodycrystalhealing.com
www.taomchi.com

UK CRYSTAL HEALING ASSOCIATIONS

Affiliation of Crystal Healing Organizations (ACHO)
PO BOX 107, Pontypool
Torfaen, Wales, NP4 4DA
www.crystal-healing.org

International Association of Crystal Healing Therapists (IACHT)
PO BOX 344, Manchester
M60 2EZ
www.iacht.co.uk

Federation of Subtle Energy Medicine
www.crystalandhealing.com

AUSTRALIAN CRYSTAL HEALING ASSOCIATIONS

The Karyna Center
T: 61 412 348 463
karyna@crystalsoundandlight.com
www.crystalsoundandlight.com

CRYSTAL SUPPLIER WEBSITES

The best way to choose crystals is to see them in person; however, if you are unable to do so, crystals can be purchased from the following sites.

US
www.bestcrystals.com
www.pelhamgrayson.com
www.crystalisinstitute.com

UK
www.crystals-online.co.uk
www.holisticshop.co.uk
www.shamanscrystal.co.uk

AUSTRALIA
www.crystalsoftheworld.com
www.hwhcrystals.com.au
www.auscrystals.com.au

INDEX

ACKNOWLEDGMENTS

Thank you to all at Ivy Press for their support and encouragement
in the creation of this book. Also thanks to all my crystal healing friends who
have shared their knowledge and enthusiasm with me over so many years.

This book is dedicated to the memory of my friend, Greta,
who gave me my first piece of amethyst more than 35 years ago.

PICTURE ACKNOWLEDGMENTS

The publisher would like to thank the Two Feathers store for their help with the photography
(www.twofeathers.co.uk), and the following for permission to reproduce copyright material:

Clipart: 101, 151, 163, 169, 209. **Alamy/**OJO Images Ltd: 35. **Bridgeman Images/**Granger: 32;
Jean Pierre Courau: 33; S. Vannini: 31. **Flickr/**Biodiversity Heritage Library: 115, 129, 211.
Ivy Press/Stephen Marwood: 67, 78, 80, 119, 166, 206; John Woodcock: 15.
Library of Congress/The H.C. Miner Litho. Co., N.Y.: 121; 133. **Shutterstock/**9photos: 150; Africa
Studio: 95; Albert Russ: 67, 77, 109, 131, 136, 200, 201, 203TR, 211; Alexander Hoffmann: 124, 175,
190; Alexander Varykhanov: 8; Anastasia Bulanova: 66T, 94, 106; Anna Lurye: 121; Aregfly: 174;
ARKHIPOV ALEKSEY: 187T; ArtofPhotos: 145; Bjoern Wylezich: 140, 184, 199, 215T; bjphotographs: 74,
153, 178B, 189, 197B; Cagla Acikgoz: 83, 181, 182; CCat82: 11; Charlie Blacker: 55; Dafinchi: 9, 79,
147, 157; dorky: 209; Elena Dijour: 175; farbled: 104, 105, 133, 134, 164; Fernando Sanchez Cortes:
129; fotoecho_com: 81; fotosaga: 25BR; Gala_Kan: 163; Grechishkin: 67, 208; gontar: 186; Gozzoli:
148; horiyan: 108; Igor Boldyrev: 98; IgorGolovniov: 95, 151, 189L; ikonacolor: 143; Ilizia: 196L; Imfoto:
79, 115, 120, 138, 185; iryna1: 141; Iurii Osadchi: 213T; J. Palys: 75, 127, 169; James L. Davidson: 13;
Jennifer Bosvert: 21T; Jianwei Zhu: 27; Jiri Vaclavek: 21B, 25TR, 210; Johannes Kornelius: 93; Karynf: 130;
klemen cerkovnik: 17; lcrms: 16; Linnas: 151; Lucie F: 91; LunarVogel: 118; Madrugada Verde: 77;
Manamana: 125B; MarcelClemens: 92, 149, 188L, 214; michaelbarrowphoto: 54L; Mivr: 87; movit: 172;
Nadezda Boltaca: 66, 82, 203B; nantarpats: 191; Nastya22: 86, 125, 159; Nika Lerman: 202; Olga
Zelenkova: 34, 58-59T; olpo: 212; Only Fabrizio: 157; Oreena: 196R; paleontologist natural: 20R; Patricia
Chumillas: 158; Pecold: 28-29; Peter Hermes Furian: 110; Phodo Design: 152, 188R; Reload Design: 103,
180; Richard Griffin: 51; Rojarin: 113; Roy Palmer: 67B, 90, 100, 102, 103, 132, 179; S_E: 67, 142;
Santhosh Varghese: 195; Sebastian Janicki: 37L; Sementer: 24R; Sergey Goryachev: 179; Sergey Lavrentev:
171; smallblackcat: 66B, 116; Stellar Gems: 146, 176; Stefan Malloch: 155; Stephen Orsillo: 76, 154;
sumire8: 24; Sundraw Photography: 25BL, 99; Tinalmages: 141; TonelloPhotography: 198; Vereschagin: 84;
Victorian Traditions: 121; vitality_73: 54R; vvoe: 25TL, 66, 67T, 85, 88, 89, 97, 101, 107, 111, 114,
117, 122, 123, 126, 128, 135, 139, 144, 156, 162, 163, 165, 168, 170, 173, 178T, 183, 187B,
192, 193, 194, 197T, 204, 205, 207, 213T; Warinezz: 199; wavebreakmedia: 2; yanikap: 20L;
yul38885: 160, 161; Yut chanthaburi: 112; Zbynek Burival: 177; Zelenskaya: 96, 97, 215B.
All other montage images courtesy of Shutterstock. **The Old Design Shop:** 187T, 121.
Wellcome Collection/William Cheselden: 115. **Wikimedia Commons/**Doris Anthony: 23;
Mirzolot2: 99, 167; Erik Hooymans: 175; Gregory H. Revera: 183.

All reasonable efforts have been made to trace copyright holders and to obtain their permission for
the use of copyright material. The publisher apologizes for any errors or omissions in the list above
and will gratefully incorporate any corrections in future reprints if notified.